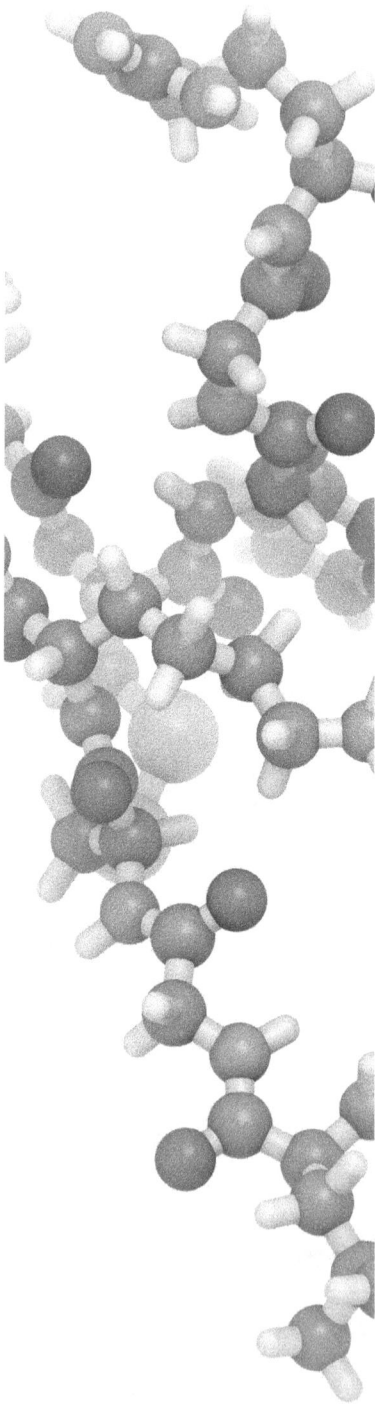

Healing with peptides: The ultimate guide to biohacking your body

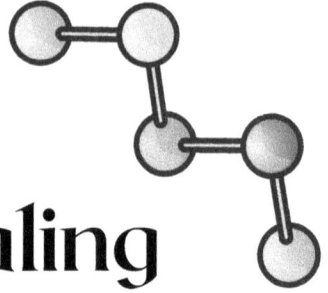

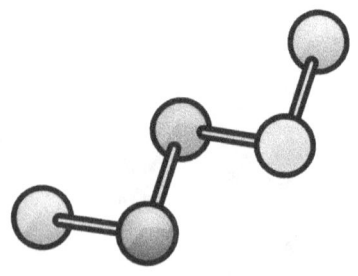

Table of Contents

Table of Contents

Introduction

It was a crisp autumn morning when I met Sarah, a vibrant 45-year-old woman who had been struggling with chronic fatigue and brain fog for years. As we sat down to discuss her health concerns, she confided in me, "I feel like I've tried everything, but nothing seems to work. I'm starting to lose hope." Little did she know her life was about to change forever.

At that moment, I knew I had to share my knowledge of peptides – the cutting-edge biohacking science that can potentially transform lives. This book, "Healing with Peptides: The Ultimate Guide to Biohacking Your Body" is my way of empowering you, just like I empowered Sarah, to take control of your health and unlock your body's innate healing potential.

Peptides, simply put, are short chains of amino acids that act as building blocks and play a crucial role in numerous biological processes. These tiny molecules are the unsung heroes of our bodies, regulating everything from metabolism and immune function to sleep and cognitive performance. By harnessing the power of peptides, we can optimize our health, enhance our vitality, and even slow down the aging process.

What sets this book apart is its commitment to making the science of peptides accessible and actionable for everyone. Whether you're a young adult looking to enhance your physical performance, an adult seeking to optimize your cognitive function better, or an elderly individual aiming to maintain your vitality, this guide will provide you with the tools and knowledge you need to succeed.

Introduction

Inside these pages, you'll discover:

- Clear, easy-to-understand definitions of peptides and their various types
- Specific protocols for using peptides to address a wide range of health concerns
- Precise dosages and administration methods for optimal results
- Real-life case studies and success stories to inspire your own journey
- Practical tips for incorporating peptides into your daily routine

As a passionate advocate for health optimization, I've dedicated my career to helping people like you achieve their highest potential, to go beyond average health to a higher level of well-being. With years of research and firsthand experience, I've witnessed the life-changing effects of peptides in countless individuals. Now, I'm thrilled to share this knowledge with you, to enable you to experience the transformative power of biohacking personally.

Throughout this book, you'll gain a deep understanding of how peptides work, why they're so effective, and how you can use them to target specific health goals. Whether you're looking to boost your energy levels, sharpen your mental focus, or enhance your overall well-being, "Healing with Peptides" will be your go-to guide.

Introduction

So, are you ready to embark on a journey of self-discovery and transformation? Are you prepared to take control of your health and unlock your body's full potential? If so, join me as we dive into the fascinating world of peptides and biohacking. Together, we'll explore cutting-edge science, uncover practical strategies, and inspire each other to live our best lives.

Let *"Healing with Peptides"* be your companion on this exciting journey. With its actionable insights, expert guidance, and inspiring stories, this book will empower you to become the architect of your own well-being.

So, turn the page, and let's begin your transformation today!

Chapter 1
Understanding the Basics of Peptides

It was during a community health workshop that I first encountered David, a retired engineer with an insatiable curiosity for the latest in health science. As he sat among a diverse group of attendees, ranging from college students to retirees, he raised a question that resonated with everyone in the room: *"What exactly are peptides, and how can they make a difference in my health?"* This inquiry set the stage for a revelation that would open up a new world of possibilities for everyone present. We live in an era where health optimization is no longer the preserve of medical professionals alone; it is a shared journey toward understanding and utilizing the many tools available to us. Peptides, often overshadowed by their larger counterparts, proteins, are emerging as pivotal players in this journey. Their simplicity and versatility make them accessible to anyone eager to enhance his or her well-being.

What Are Peptides? A Non-Scientist's Explanation

Peptides, in their essence, are short chains of amino acids, the very building blocks of life. Imagine constructing a house; peptides are akin to the bricks used to form the structure. They are smaller than proteins, consisting of no more than 50 amino acids, which makes them remarkably straightforward yet incredibly diverse in function. While proteins are complex and often intimidating to those without a scientific background, peptides offer a more approachable introduction to the world of biochemistry. Their role as signaling molecules highlights their importance in regulating essential physiological processes. They act as messengers, transmitting vital information throughout the body, and influencing everything from how we metabolize food to how we respond to stress.

In the realm of biological processes, peptides hold a position of great significance. They are integral in signaling pathways, akin to the way traffic lights direct the flow of vehicles. This signaling ensures that our body functions smoothly, maintaining balance and harmony within our complex systems.

Take insulin, for example, a peptide hormone that plays a crucial role in regulating blood sugar levels. Without insulin, our body's ability to manage glucose effectively would be compromised, leading to serious health issues. Similarly, collagen peptides contribute to the strength and elasticity of our connective tissues, supporting skin, bones, and joints. These examples illustrate how deeply embedded peptides are in our everyday lives, and they offer a glimpse into their vast potential for promoting and elevating health and wellness.

Peptides occur naturally in the body and are also found in various foods that we consume – or should be consuming. They are present in dairy products like milk and cheese, and in meat like chicken and fish, providing us with the amino acids essential for building and repairing tissues. This natural abundance underscores their role as fundamental components of our diet and physiology. The simplicity of peptides compared to proteins is one of their most appealing attributes.

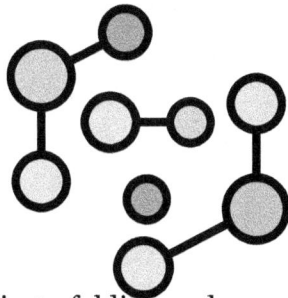

Proteins, with their intricate folding and complex structures, can often seem daunting. Peptides, however, offer a more straightforward approach to understanding the biochemical mechanisms that govern our health. This simplicity makes them ideal candidates for biohacking, where precision and specificity are key. By biohacking, we mean individuals working on their own to improve their physical and mental performance.

The beauty of peptides lies not only in their simplicity but also in their versatility. Their ability to adapt and perform various functions within the body makes them invaluable tools for health optimization. Whether you are a young adult looking to boost your physical performance, an adult seeking cognitive enhancement, or an elderly individual aiming to maintain vitality, peptides offer practical solutions tailored to meet diverse needs.

As we explore the fascinating world of peptides in this book, you'll discover actionable insights and practical applications that are easily implemented in your daily life. From understanding specific peptide functions to learning about precise dosages and administration methods, this guide is designed to empower you with the knowledge needed to take control of your health.

- **In this chapter, we will delve deeper into what makes peptides such a powerful tool in the quest for optimal wellness.**

You'll gain a clearer understanding of their fundamental role in our bodies and learn how to leverage their potential to achieve your health goals. With this foundation, you'll be well-equipped to explore the subsequent chapters, where we'll uncover specific applications and benefits of peptides across various aspects of health. The journey ahead promises to be enlightening, offering new insights and possibilities for enhancing your well-being through the remarkable world of peptides.

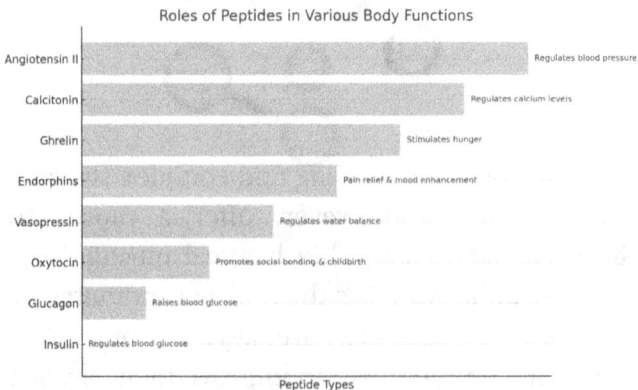

Roles of Peptides in Various Body Functions

Peptide Types	
Angiotensin II	Regulates blood pressure
Calcitonin	Regulates calcium levels
Ghrelin	Stimulates hunger
Endorphins	Pain relief & mood enhancement
Vasopressin	Regulates water balance
Oxytocin	Promotes social bonding & childbirth
Glucagon	Raises blood glucose
Insulin	Regulates blood glucose

The Science of Peptides: Cellular Functions and Interactions

Imagine a bustling corporation where messages are constantly exchanged to keep everything running smoothly. This corporation is your body, and the messengers are peptides. At the cellular level, peptides perform a crucial role akin to skilled diplomats, navigating through complex pathways to deliver their messages accurately. They achieve this by binding to specific receptors embedded in cell membranes, much like a key fitting into a lock. This interaction initiates a cascade of signaling events within the cell, triggering responses that are fundamental to maintaining health. The beauty of this system lies in its precision — each peptide and receptor pair is designed to interact precisely, ensuring that messages are delivered only where needed.

Once a peptide binds to its receptor, it activates intracellular signaling pathways, which are akin to a series of interconnected roads leading to various destinations within the cell. These pathways facilitate communication and coordination, allowing the cell to respond appropriately to external and internal cues. For example, when a peptide involved in metabolism binds to its receptor, it may activate pathways that influence how the cell processes nutrients. Through these pathways, peptides can modulate a myriad of cellular activities, from growth and repair to immune responses and hormone production.

Peptides also play a pivotal role in facilitating intercellular communication, acting as the body's very own postal service – or mailroom. In neurotransmission, for instance, peptides help transmit signals across synapses, the small gaps between nerve cells. This process is essential for brain function, affecting everything from mood and memory to movement and sensation. Similarly, in hormone signaling, peptides serve as messengers that relay information between glands and target organs, orchestrating processes that regulate growth, metabolism, and stress responses. Their ability to transmit signals efficiently and accurately is what makes peptides indispensable in the realm of cellular communication.

One of the most intriguing aspects of peptides is their ability to influence gene expression, a process akin to editing the script of a play. By interacting with specific transcription factors and DNA sequences, peptides can modulate which genes are turned on or off, thereby influencing protein synthesis. This control over gene expression allows peptides to regulate metabolic pathways and adapt cellular functions to changing conditions. For instance, a peptide might upgrade the production of enzymes involved in energy metabolism during times of high physical activity, ensuring that the body has sufficient fuel to meet increased demands.

Scientific research provides a robust foundation for understanding peptide functions. Studies have shown that targeting peptide-mediated interactions can offer therapeutic benefits, such as drug development and disease therapy (Source 3). By exploring these interactions, researchers have identified numerous applications for peptides, ranging from treating metabolic disorders to enhancing cognitive function. The versatility of peptides in influencing cellular processes highlights their potential as powerful tools for health optimization. As we continue to unravel the complexities of peptide interactions, new opportunities for therapeutic interventions and biohacking strategies will undoubtedly emerge.

In essence, peptides operate as dynamic contributors to cellular communication and function, their actions integral to the harmonious operation of our biological systems. Whether through signaling pathways, gene expression, or intercellular communication, peptides exemplify the intricate interplay of molecules that sustain life. Understanding these mechanisms not only enriches our knowledge of biology but also empowers us to harness the potential power of peptides in enhancing our health and well-being. As we navigate the fascinating landscape of peptide science, we uncover not only the intricacies of our own biology but also the possibilities for innovation in health and medicine.

Peptide Categories and Their Unique Properties

When considering the vast world of peptides, it becomes evident that categorizing them based on function allows for a more organized and practical understanding. Among the most significant categories are hormonal peptides, which include well-known examples like growth hormone. These peptides are vital in regulating metabolism, acting much like conductors in an orchestra, ensuring that each section performs its role in harmony.

They influence how our bodies utilize energy, manage stress, and even regulate growth and reproductive functions. Due to their pivotal role, hormonal peptides are often at the forefront of therapeutic applications, offering potential treatments for conditions like growth deficiencies and metabolic disorders.

Another essential category is neurotransmitter peptides, such as endorphins, which play a crucial role in communication within the nervous system. Endorphins, often dubbed the body's natural painkillers, are released in response to stress or discomfort, helping alleviate pain and enhance feelings of pleasure. Their impact on mood and emotional well-being makes them invaluable in addressing mental health issues, such as depression and anxiety, highlighting the therapeutic potential of neurotransmitter peptides.

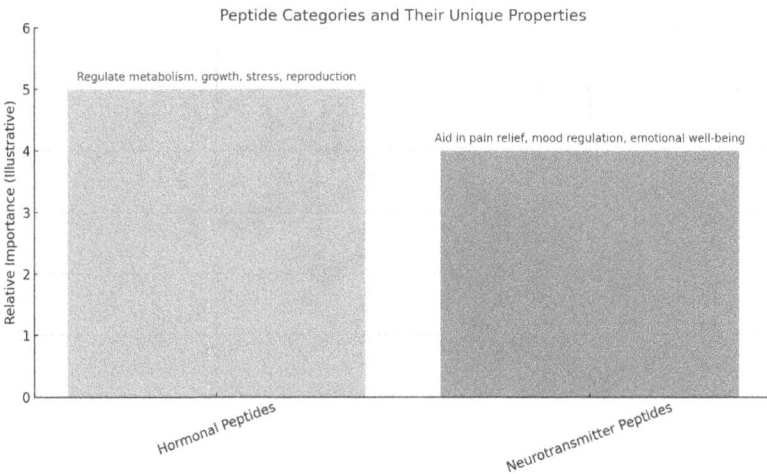

Peptide Categories and Their Unique Properties

The uniqueness of peptide categories lies in their distinct properties and their specific roles in health maintenance. Hormonal peptides, for example, can modulate metabolic pathways, adjust energy expenditure, and maintain homeostasis. This regulatory function is crucial in preventing metabolic imbalances that can lead to obesity, diabetes, and other chronic conditions. On the other hand, antimicrobial peptides serve as the body's defenders against invading pathogens. These peptides utilize their protective properties by disrupting the membranes of bacteria, viruses, and fungi, providing a first line of defense in the immune response.

Their potential as alternatives to traditional antibiotics is of great interest, especially in the face of rising antibiotic resistance. The diversity of peptide functions extends further, encompassing roles in immune response, cellular repair, and maintenance. Peptides involved in immune response act as sentinels, identifying and neutralizing threats before they compromise our health. They stimulate the production of antibodies, enhance the activity of immune cells, and promote the clearance of pathogens.

In cellular repair and maintenance, peptides facilitate the regeneration of damaged tissues, supporting healing and recovery. Their ability to promote collagen production, for instance, aids skin repair and the maintenance of joint health, making them popular in cosmetic and orthopedic applications.

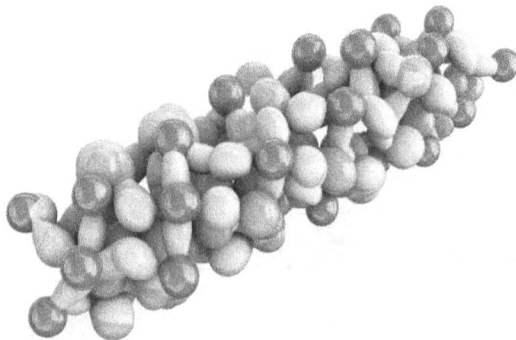

The versatility of peptides is a testament to their adaptability and wide-ranging applications in health and disease. Each category of peptides serves multiple roles, adapting to the body's needs and providing targeted interventions. Peptides in the immune response, for instance, protect against infections as well as modulate inflammation, a process that, when left uncontrolled, can lead to chronic diseases.

Similarly, peptides involved in cellular repair contribute to tissue regeneration and recovery, making them valuable in treating injuries and degenerative conditions. By categorizing peptides based on their functions, we can better appreciate their therapeutic uses in biohacking and beyond.

This classification guides the development of peptide-based therapies, allowing for tailored interventions that address specific health concerns. Hormonal peptides, with their metabolic regulatory capabilities, offer promising solutions for weight management, diabetes, and hormone replacement therapies. Antimicrobial peptides provide alternatives in infection control and immune support, while neurotransmitter peptides offer new avenues for managing mood disorders and enhancing cognitive function.

In understanding these categories, we unlock the potential to harness peptides' unique properties for health optimization. By aligning peptide functions with therapeutic applications, we can develop personalized strategies that leverage their strengths, ultimately enhancing well-being and preventing disease. This knowledge empowers individuals to make informed choices about their health as they utilize peptides as tools in their pursuit of optimal wellness.

As we explore the fascinating diversity of peptides, we uncover opportunities to innovate in health care, pave the way for new treatments, and interventions that capitalize on the remarkable properties of these versatile molecules.

Peptides vs. Proteins: Understanding the Distinctions

In the vibrant tapestry of biological molecules, proteins stand out as the architects of life, weaving together the intricate patterns of existence.

- These molecules, long chains of amino acids, fold into complex structures that determine their diverse functions.
- Proteins can be likened to the intricate blueprints of a skyscraper, each fold and twist critical to maintaining the structure's integrity and function.
- Meanwhile, peptides, often precursors to these larger proteins, are the simpler artisans, crafting specific components essential for the body's immediate needs.
- With typically fewer than 50 amino acids, peptides are more focused on their roles, offering specific, targeted actions within the cellular milieu.
- This distinction between the long chains of proteins and the shorter sequences of peptides is foundational, affecting everything from their biological roles to their therapeutic applications.

The complexity of *proteins* arises from their ability to fold into secondary, tertiary, and quaternary structures. This folding is like a masterful origami artist transforming a simple piece of paper into a three-dimensional work of art. Each fold in a protein serves a specific purpose, often creating binding sites that allow proteins to interact with other molecules. This complexity enables proteins to serve as enzymes catalyzing biochemical reactions, structural components providing support and shape to cells, and transporters ferrying molecules across cellular membranes.

In contrast, *peptides*, with their simpler, linear structures, act with precision and specificity, binding to receptors or interacting with other molecules to trigger specific responses. Their simplicity allows peptides to act swiftly and effectively, making them ideal for regulatory roles within the body.

Both peptides and proteins contribute significantly to biological diversity, each playing unique roles in maintaining the body's homeostasis. Proteins, with their vast range of functions, are the workhorses of all cells. They perform tasks ranging from catalyzing metabolic reactions to serving as the scaffolding that maintains cell shape.

Meanwhile, peptides function as versatile regulatory molecules, orchestrating processes such as cell signaling and immune responses. Imagine a bustling city where proteins are the infrastructure—buildings, roads, bridges—providing the city with its physical form and function. Peptides, in this analogy, are the city's communication network, ensuring that information flows smoothly, directing traffic, and coordinating responses to various stimuli.

The practical implications of these differences are profound, influencing how we utilize peptides and proteins in therapies and biohacking strategies. In medical treatments, proteins often serve as replacement therapies, such as insulin for diabetes. Their complex structures allow them to replace or augment natural proteins that may be deficient or malfunctioning.

However, the complexity of proteins also presents challenges, such as potential immunogenicity and the need for specific delivery methods to ensure stability and activity. Peptides, with their simpler structures, offer distinct advantages. They can be designed to target specific receptors, providing precise interventions with minimal side effects. Their ability to be synthesized and modified easily makes them attractive candidates for developing novel therapies, from targeting cancer cells to modulating immune responses.

- In the realm of biohacking, these distinctions allow for innovative approaches to health optimization.
- Peptides can be tailored to enhance specific physiological functions, offering targeted solutions for everything from improving sleep quality to boosting cognitive performance.
- Their specificity reduces the risk of unintended effects, a critical consideration for those seeking to fine-tune their biology safely.
- Meanwhile, proteins, with their multifunctional capabilities, provide foundational support, ensuring the body's systems operate efficiently.
- The balance between these molecules is akin to a well-coordinated orchestra, where each instrument plays its part, and only its part, thus contributing to the harmony of the whole.
- Understanding these distinctions not only deepens our appreciation for the complexity of life but also empowers us to leverage these molecules in our quest for better health and enhanced vitality.

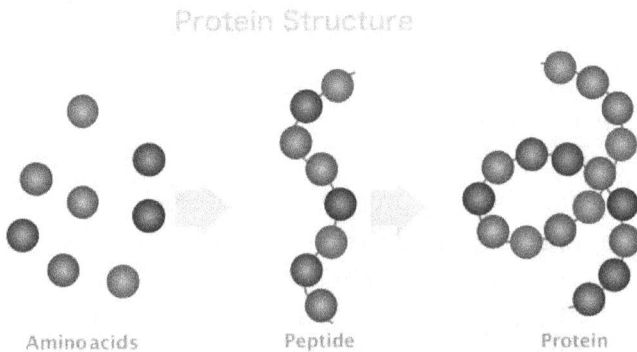

Protein Structure

Amino acids   Peptide   Protein

The Endocrine System and Peptides: A Synergistic Relationship

In the intricate dance of the human body, the endocrine system plays a pivotal role as the conductor, orchestrating a symphony of hormones that regulate vital functions. One of its key players are peptides, which act as hormones to ensure that every process runs smoothly. Imagine peptides as the notes in a melody, each contributing to the harmony of growth, metabolism, and reproduction. Their influence is profound, guiding the body's development and energy management.

For instance, growth hormone, a peptide, is crucial during childhood and adolescence, fueling growth and cell reproduction. As we age, it helps maintain muscle mass and bone density, illustrating its lifelong importance. Meanwhile, other peptides regulate metabolism, ensuring that our bodies efficiently convert food into energy. This process is akin to a well-tuned engine, running seamlessly to power our daily activities. In the realm of reproduction, peptides also take center stage, influencing the release of hormones that govern fertility and sexual function. They ensure the delicate balance necessary for these complex processes to occur, demonstrating their indispensable role in life's continuity.

GROWTH HORMONE

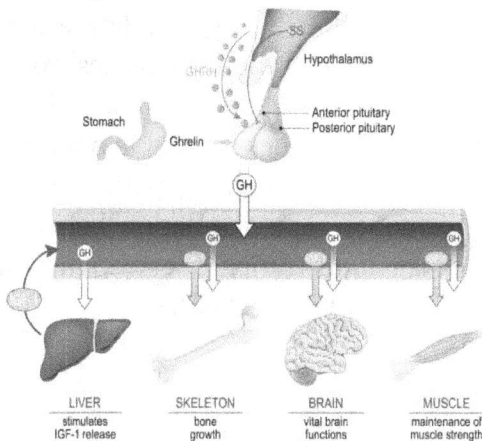

The integration of peptides with hormones within the endocrine system is a testament to the body's remarkable complexity. Insulin, a well-known peptide hormone, exemplifies this synergy by managing glucose metabolism. Like a diligent accountant, insulin ensures that blood sugar levels remain stable, distributing glucose to cells for energy or storing it for later use. This regulation prevents the extreme effects of hyperglycemia and hypoglycemia, protecting the body from potential damage. Similarly, glucagon, another peptide hormone, acts as insulin's counterpart, raising blood sugar levels when they drop too low.

This dynamic duo exemplifies the balance that peptides and hormones maintain, a fine-tuned system of checks and balances that safeguards our health. Such interactions highlight the precise and coordinated nature of peptide action, reinforcing their importance in the endocrine system's regulatory framework.

Peptides are also integral to feedback mechanisms within the endocrine system, ensuring that the body's internal environment remains stable. These feedback loops operate like a thermostat, adjusting hormone levels to maintain equilibrium. In negative feedback loops, an increase in a particular hormone signals the body to reduce its production, preventing excess.

This mechanism is crucial in hormone regulation by preventing imbalances that could lead to disorders. For example, when blood sugar levels rise, insulin secretion increases to facilitate glucose acceptance by cells. Once equilibrium is restored, insulin production decreases, illustrating the feedback loop in action. Peptides also play a role in stress response, with signaling pathways that modulate the release of stress hormones. This regulation helps the body adapt to changing conditions, demonstrating the dynamic nature of peptide involvement in maintaining homeostasis.

The implications of understanding peptides within the endocrine system extend into the realm of biohacking, offering promising avenues for health optimization. By leveraging peptide knowledge, individuals can address hormonal imbalances through targeted therapies. These interventions can help regulate thyroid function, support adrenal health, and manage other endocrine disorders, providing a holistic approach to well-being. Furthermore, optimizing metabolic processes through peptide use can enhance energy levels, support weight management, and improve overall vitality. This application is particularly relevant in today's fast-paced world, where maintaining optimal health has never been more challenging or necessary. As we continue to explore the potential of peptides in the endocrine system, we unlock new possibilities for personalized medicine and biohacking strategies. This understanding empowers us to take charge of our health, utilizing the body's natural mechanisms to achieve balance and vitality.

The synergy between peptides and the endocrine system is not just a marvel of biology; instead, it is a gateway to innovative approaches to health and wellness.

Common Misconceptions about Peptides Debunked

In the realm of health and wellness, misconceptions often cloud the true potential of peptides, leaving many wary of their use. One prevalent myth is the concern over their safety and efficacy. The reality is that peptides boast a strong safety profile in therapeutic settings, largely due to their natural role in the body. When administered correctly, peptides rarely cause severe side effects. Most issues arise from improper use or sourcing from unreliable suppliers.

Thus, understanding the source and ensuring proper dosage are key to safe usage. Minor side effects, like irritation at injection sites, tend to be temporary and manageable. This contrasts starkly with the exaggerated fears perpetuated by misinformation.

Further complicating the conversation is the misunderstanding surrounding the legality of peptide use. Many assume peptides are unregulated or illegal. In truth, peptide use is legal when appropriately prescribed by a healthcare provider.

However, purchasing peptides from unverified online sources can pose legal and health risks. These products might not meet safety standards, leading to potential legal consequences. It's crucial to understand that while peptides are accessible, their use should be guided by medical advice.

Ethical considerations also play a role, particularly in research. Ensuring informed consent and transparency is vital to maintaining ethical standards in peptide studies. These principles safeguard participants and uphold the integrity of scientific exploration.

Another area of confusion involves the capabilities of peptides. Some believe peptides are miracle cures for a plethora of ailments. While they hold immense potential, peptides are not a panacea. They offer targeted benefits, but their efficacy depends on the specific peptide and condition being treated. For instance, while some peptides can aid in muscle growth or fat loss, they require lifestyle changes to maximize their effects. Overhyping peptide abilities can lead to unrealistic expectations. It's important to approach peptide use with a nuanced understanding of their benefits and limitations. Recognizing these boundaries helps set realistic health goals and ensures a balanced approach to wellness.

To counter these myths, we turn to scientific evidence and expert insights. Studies consistently show that when used properly, peptides can significantly enhance health outcomes. For example, research highlights their role in improving metabolic function and supporting tissue repair. These findings are backed by rigorous clinical trials that adhere to strict ethical guidelines. Additionally, expert opinions reinforce the importance of informed peptide use. They emphasize the need for professional guidance and the benefits of integrating peptides into a broader health and lifestyle strategy. By relying on credible sources, we can dispel misinformation and make informed decisions about peptide use.

Peptides, when used correctly, offer a promising avenue for health optimization. Addressing common misconceptions allows us to appreciate their true value without the distortion of myths. As we continue to explore the potential of peptides, it's essential to ground our understanding in facts. This approach not only enhances our knowledge but powers us to use peptides effectively and responsibly. By embracing a balanced perspective, we can integrate peptides into our wellness routines with confidence. The journey to health optimization is filled with opportunities, and peptides are valuable tools in this pursuit. Let us move forward with clarity and purpose, ensuring our understanding of peptides is informed and accurate.

Chapter 2
Diving into the Mechanisms
of Action

Imagine your body as a complex orchestra, where each cell plays a specific instrument, guided by the maestro of biochemical signals. Among these signals are peptides, the maestros of cellular communication, orchestrating symphonies of reactions and responses. Consider a scenario where you're beginning a new workout routine. You might notice how your body adapts to increased physical demands, building endurance and strength over time. Behind this transformation are peptides, orchestrating cellular changes, enhancing muscle repair, and optimizing energy use. This chapter unravels the intricacies of how peptides influence such transformations, revealing the magic behind their ability to modulate our biological symphony.

At the heart of peptide action are signaling pathways, intricate networks that dictate cellular behavior. These pathways are like digital highways, transmitting signals that instruct cells how to respond to changes. Peptides play a crucial role in activating these pathways, often acting as the initial signal or ligand. Upon binding to a receptor, a peptide triggers a cascade of intracellular events, akin to a series of falling dominos. One of the primary mechanisms through which peptides exert their effects is the activation of secondary messenger systems. These systems amplify the initial signal, ensuring that the message is broadcast throughout the cell.

For example, cyclic AMP (cAMP) is a common secondary messenger that mediates numerous cellular processes, from energy balance to hormone secretion. This amplification allows even a small number of peptide molecules to elicit a significant physiological response, demonstrating their efficiency and potency.

The molecular basis of peptide action is rooted in their chemical interactions, particularly their binding affinity and specificity. This interaction is akin to a lock-and-key mechanism, where the peptide is the key that fits precisely into the receptor's lock. This specificity ensures that peptides only activate their intended targets, minimizing unintended effects. Binding affinity, on the other hand, refers to the strength of this interaction. A peptide with high affinity binds more tightly to its receptor, resulting in a more prolonged and potent effect. This precise interaction allows peptides to modulate biological processes with such accuracy.

For example, in the regulation of metabolic rates, peptides like glucagon-like peptide-1 (GLP-1) bind to receptors on pancreatic cells to enhance insulin secretion, thereby controlling blood sugar levels. Similarly, peptides can influence circadian rhythms, the body's internal clock, by interacting with receptors in the brain that regulate sleep-wake cycles. This modulation highlights the diverse roles peptides play in maintaining physiological balance and adapting to environmental cues.

Glucagon-like peptide-1

GLP-1

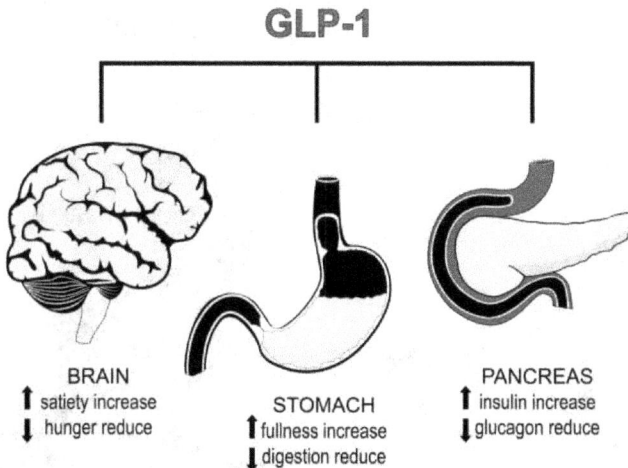

BRAIN
↑ satiety increase
↓ hunger reduce

STOMACH
↑ fullness increase
↓ digestion reduce

PANCREAS
↑ insulin increase
↓ glucagon reduce

The implications of peptide mechanisms extend into therapeutic realms, offering promising avenues for treating various health conditions. In metabolic disorders like type 2 diabetes, peptides such as GLP-1 analogs are used to improve insulin sensitivity and glycemic control, providing a targeted approach to managing the disease (Source 3). These therapies capitalize on the natural mechanisms of peptide action, enhancing the body's ability to regulate blood sugar levels. In regenerative medicine, peptides are explored for their potential to promote tissue repair and regeneration. By modulating growth factors and signaling pathways, peptides can accelerate healing processes, offering hope for conditions ranging from chronic wounds to degenerative diseases. The targeted nature of peptide therapies ensures that they can deliver benefits with minimal side effects, enhancing their appeal as a treatment option.

As we delve deeper into the mechanisms of peptide action, the potential for innovation and discovery becomes evident. Peptides offer a unique lens through which we can view and manipulate biological systems, providing insights into the fundamental processes that underlie health and disease. Their ability to precisely modulate cellular functions opens new possibilities for therapeutic interventions, promising a future where treatments are not only effective but also tailored to individual needs. The understanding of peptide mechanisms is not just a scientific endeavor; it is a gateway to improving human health in profound ways.

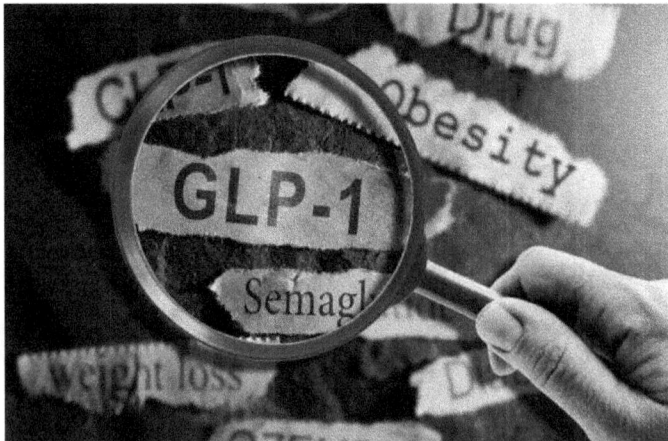

Cellular Receptors and Peptides: A Complex Interaction

Imagine your body as a bustling city, where peptides are like specialized couriers delivering vital messages. For these messages to reach their destination, they must interact with specific receptors on cell surfaces. These receptors are like the mailboxes of the cellular world, designed to receive only specific types of mail. Among the most important receptors that peptides interact with are G-protein coupled receptors (GPCRs) and tyrosine kinase receptors. GPCRs are incredibly versatile and are involved in nearly every physiological process. They possess a unique ability to undergo conformational changes when a peptide binds, triggering a cascade of intracellular events.

Tyrosine kinase receptors, on the other hand, are primarily involved in growth and differentiation. When a peptide binds to these receptors, it often leads to the activation of pathways that control cell division and survival. These receptors are crucial for processes such as wound healing and immune responses.

The interaction between peptides and receptors is a finely tuned process, marked by specificity and selectivity. Picture a lock and key, where the peptide is the key that fits precisely into the receptor lock. This specificity ensures that each peptide binds only to its designated receptor, triggering the appropriate response. The conformation of the receptor, or its three-dimensional shape, plays a pivotal role in this interaction. When a peptide binds, the receptor changes its shape, which is essential for activating downstream signaling pathways. This change is akin to flipping a switch that sets off a series of reactions within the cell. The high selectivity of this binding means that even slight variations in the peptide structure can affect its ability to bind, highlighting the precision of these biological interactions.

Once a peptide binds to a receptor, it initiates a series of cellular responses that are both immediate and far-reaching. This interaction triggers signal transduction pathways, complex networks of molecules that communicate signals from the cell surface to the interior. These pathways are like relay races, where each molecule passes the baton to the next, amplifying the signal as it moves along. One well-known pathway is the mitogen-activated protein kinase (MAPK) pathway, which plays a significant role in cell growth and survival. Another is the phosphoinositide 3-kinase (PI3K) pathway, involved in metabolism and cell survival. Beyond immediate signaling, peptide-receptor interactions can also modulate gene expression, influencing which genes are turned on or off. This modulation is crucial for long-term cellular responses, such as differentiation and adaptation to environmental changes.

Understanding these intricate interactions has profound implications for drug development. By elucidating the dynamics of peptide-receptor binding, researchers can design more effective peptide-based therapies. This knowledge allows for the creation of drugs that mimic or block natural peptide functions, offering targeted treatments with fewer side effects. The specificity of peptide-receptor interactions makes them ideal candidates for precision medicine, where therapies are tailored to individual needs. For instance, in cancer treatment, drugs targeting specific tyrosine kinase receptors can inhibit tumor growth by blocking the signals that promote cell division. Similarly, GPCR-targeted therapies have shown promise in treating conditions like heart disease and mental health disorders. By leveraging our understanding of these interactions, we can develop innovative therapies that address a wide range of health challenges, from metabolic disorders to autoimmune diseases.

Peptides and Homeostasis: Achieving Balance in the Body

Imagine trying to keep a seesaw perfectly balanced, where every slight movement requires a counterbalance to maintain equilibrium. This is much like the concept of homeostasis in the human body. Homeostasis refers to the body's ability to maintain a stable internal environment despite external changes. It's why your body temperature remains relatively constant even when the weather shifts from a scorching summer afternoon to a chilly winter night.

Achieving this balance is crucial for health, as every cell, tissue, and organ functions optimally within a narrow range of conditions. Disruptions can lead to disease, making the maintenance of homeostasis fundamental to well-being. Imagine it as the body's own thermostat, constantly adjusting to keep everything running smoothly.

Peptides play a pivotal role in maintaining this balance, acting as regulators across various physiological systems. For instance, in temperature regulation, certain peptides help the body adjust to fluctuations, ensuring that enzymes and metabolic processes operate efficiently. Consider a day spent outdoors; whether you're sweating under the sun or shivering in the cold, peptides signal sweat glands to cool you down or muscles to generate heat through shivering.

Similarly, peptides manage fluid and electrolyte balance, which is crucial for cellular function. They signal the kidneys to adjust water reabsorption, ensuring hydration levels are optimal and that electrolytes like sodium and potassium are in harmony. This regulation is vital, as imbalances can affect everything from nerve transmission to heart function.

Feedback mechanisms are key to how peptides maintain homeostasis. Think of them as intricate feedback loops, like a thermostat adjusting a heating system. Peptides regulate hunger and satiety signals, ensuring energy intake matches expenditure. When you eat a meal, peptides like ghrelin and leptin communicate with the brain to signal fullness or hunger, guiding your food intake. This system prevents overeating and ensures energy reserves are maintained. Such feedback loops are essential in preventing metabolic disorders like obesity and diabetes, which arise from imbalances in these signals. Peptides act as messengers, conveying information about the body's status and prompting necessary adjustments.

In conditions where homeostasis is disrupted, peptides offer therapeutic potential to restore balance. For instance, in diseased states like heart failure or chronic dehydration, peptide-based treatments can be designed to correct imbalances. By mimicking or enhancing natural peptide actions, these therapies can support the body's efforts to regain equilibrium. In heart failure, peptides that promote vasodilation and reduce fluid retention can alleviate symptoms and improve quality of life. Similarly, in conditions like hyponatremia, where sodium levels are too low, peptides can help regulate kidney function to restore balance. These interventions highlight the potential of peptides not just in maintaining health but in correcting dysregulation when it occurs.

Understanding the role of peptides in homeostasis underscores their importance in both health and disease. They act as the body's natural regulators, ensuring stability in the face of change. By modulating various physiological processes, peptides help maintain the delicate balance that is essential for life. This knowledge opens doors to innovative treatments that harness the power of peptides to restore balance in diseased states, offering hope for conditions where traditional therapies may fall short. As we continue to explore the potential of peptides, their role in achieving and maintaining homeostasis remains a cornerstone of their therapeutic promise.

Peptides and the Nervous System: Enhancing Cognitive Function

Envision the brain as a bustling network of highways, where neurotransmitters act as vehicles carrying vital information. In this intricate system, peptides function as specialized conductors, fine-tuning the speed and direction of these vehicles. By facilitating synaptic transmission, peptides enhance the communication between neurons, ensuring that messages travel swiftly and accurately across synapses. This enhanced communication is critical for everything from reflexive actions to complex decision-making processes. For instance, peptides can modulate the release of neurotransmitters such as dopamine and serotonin, which play pivotal roles in mood regulation and reward-driven behaviors. Through such interactions, peptides support a fluid and efficient nervous system, paving the way for sharper cognitive abilities and emotional stability.

The potential of peptides to boost mental performance is an exciting frontier in the world of cognitive enhancement. Certain peptides are known to enhance memory, a crucial aspect of learning and retaining information. They achieve this by promoting synaptic plasticity, the brain's ability to strengthen or weaken connections between neurons in response to new information. This plasticity is the foundation for learning and memory formation. Peptides like Noopept and Cerebrolysin have shown promise in enhancing cognitive processes by supporting synaptic function and increasing neurotrophic factors that foster neuron growth and survival. These peptides not only aid in memory retention but also enhance focus and concentration, critical components for productivity in daily life. By optimizing these cognitive functions, peptides offer the potential for improved mental clarity and efficiency, making them appealing to individuals seeking to enhance their cognitive capabilities.

Beyond boosting cognitive function, peptides also possess neuroprotective properties that shield the brain from age-related decline and neurodegenerative diseases. This protective effect is particularly relevant in the context of diseases like Alzheimer's and Parkinson's, where neuronal damage and loss are prevalent. Peptides can mitigate such damage by reducing oxidative stress and inflammation, which are key contributors to neuronal degeneration. For instance, peptides that mimic the action of nerve growth factors can promote the survival and repair of neurons, offering a potential therapeutic avenue for neurodegenerative conditions. By bolstering the brain's natural defenses, peptides protect against cognitive decline and support overall brain health, ensuring that cognitive functions remain robust throughout life.

In addition to their cognitive and protective roles, peptides significantly influence mood regulation. The balance of neurotransmitters in the brain directly impacts emotional states, and peptides play an integral role in maintaining this balance. Peptides like oxytocin, often referred to as the "love hormone," enhance feelings of trust and bonding, promoting positive social interactions and emotional well-being. Other peptides, such as Selank, have demonstrated anxiolytic properties, reducing anxiety by modulating the release of stress hormones and neurotransmitters. By influencing these chemical messengers, peptides can alleviate symptoms of anxiety and depression, fostering a sense of calm and stability. This makes them valuable tools in managing mood disorders and enhancing emotional resilience, offering a natural approach to achieving mental wellness.

Peptides, with their multifaceted roles in neurotransmission, cognitive enhancement, neuroprotection, and mood regulation, present a compelling case for their integration into strategies aimed at optimizing brain health. They empower individuals to take proactive steps in enhancing cognitive function that protect against decline and fostering emotional well-being. As research continues to uncover the vast potential of peptides in the nervous system, their application in enhancing mental performance and well-being becomes increasingly promising.

The Role of Peptides in Muscle Synthesis and Repair

When you think of building muscle, images of lifting weights and protein shakes might come to mind. However, beneath the surface, it's peptides that play a pivotal role in muscle growth and repair. Among these, growth hormone-releasing peptides (GHRPs) are particularly notable. These peptides stimulate the pituitary gland to release growth hormone, a key player in muscle anabolism. Growth hormone acts much like a foreman on a construction site, orchestrating the building and repair of muscle tissues. It enhances protein synthesis, which is crucial for muscle growth. Proteins serve as the bricks and mortar, while peptides ensure that these building materials are efficiently utilized to construct stronger, larger muscles.

Muscle repair is an intricate process that involves restoring damaged tissue, often due to exercise-induced microtears. Peptides facilitate this repair by promoting protein synthesis, ensuring that new proteins are produced to replace damaged ones. This process is akin to a diligent repair crew fixing a road after heavy traffic has caused wear and tear. Peptides also play a role in reducing muscle catabolism, the breakdown of muscle proteins for energy. By minimizing this breakdown, peptides help preserve muscle mass and accelerate recovery. This dual action of promoting synthesis while reducing degradation allows for more rapid and effective muscle repair, crucial for anyone engaged in regular physical activity.

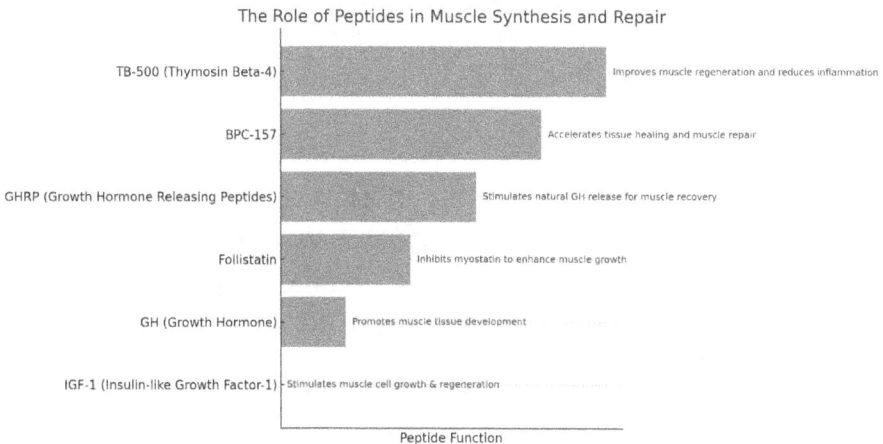

The Role of Peptides in Muscle Synthesis and Repair

Peptide	Function
TB-500 (Thymosin Beta-4)	Improves muscle regeneration and reduces inflammation
BPC-157	Accelerates tissue healing and muscle repair
GHRP (Growth Hormone Releasing Peptides)	Stimulates natural GH release for muscle recovery
Follistatin	Inhibits myostatin to enhance muscle growth
GH (Growth Hormone)	Promotes muscle tissue development
IGF-1 (Insulin-like Growth Factor-1)	Stimulates muscle cell growth & regeneration

Peptide Function

For athletes and fitness enthusiasts, peptides offer potential enhancements in performance by taking them to an even higher level. They not only aid in muscle growth but also improve endurance. Certain peptides enhance the body's ability to utilize oxygen and nutrients, boosting stamina and delaying fatigue. Imagine running a marathon; peptides can be the difference between hitting the wall and crossing the finish line with energy to spare. They optimize cellular energy production, enabling muscles to perform at their peak for longer periods. This is particularly beneficial for endurance athletes who rely on sustained energy output to excel in their sports. The ability of peptides to enhance both strength and endurance makes them a valuable asset in the world of athletic performance.

Beyond the realm of sports, peptides hold significant promise in rehabilitation. Injuries, whether from sports or daily activities, often require a period of recovery and repair. Peptides can accelerate this process by promoting tissue regeneration and reducing inflammation. Consider an athlete who has suffered a torn ligament. Peptide therapy can facilitate faster healing, allowing for a quicker return to activity. This therapeutic use is not limited to athletes; anyone recovering from surgery or injury can benefit from the regenerative properties of peptides. By enhancing the body's natural repair mechanisms, peptides support a more efficient and complete recovery, reducing downtime and improving overall outcomes.

In understanding the multifaceted roles of peptides in muscle synthesis and repair, it becomes clear that they are more than just supplements; they are integral components of the body's ability to grow, repair, and perform. Their applications extend beyond the gym, offering therapeutic benefits in injury recovery and rehabilitation. Whether you're an athlete looking to boost performance or someone recovering from an injury, peptides provide valuable tools for enhancing muscle health and function. Their ability to stimulate growth, repair tissue, and improve endurance positions them as key players in the pursuit of physical excellence and recovery.

Peptides in the Regulation of Inflammation and Immunity

Imagine your immune system as a vigilant security team, always on the lookout for intruders and ready to spring into action when a threat is detected. Peptides act as crucial members of this team, modulating immune responses to ensure that they are both effective and balanced. Peptides can serve as immunostimulants, enhancing the activity of the immune system when a robust response is needed. For example, during an infection, certain peptides can boost the production of white blood cells, the body's primary defenders against pathogens. This enhanced immune response helps to swiftly neutralize threats, preventing them from causing harm.

Furthermore, peptides play a significant role in regulating inflammation, a natural response to injury or infection that can become problematic if left unchecked. Inflammation is like a fire alarm system; it alerts the body to danger, but if the alarm blares continuously, it can lead to greater damage. Peptides help regulate this process by influencing cytokines, proteins that act as messengers in the immune system. By modulating cytokine levels, peptides can reduce excessive inflammation and promote healing.

Certain peptides inhibit pro-inflammatory mediators, effectively dampening the inflammatory response. This action can be particularly beneficial in conditions characterized by chronic inflammation, such as arthritis, where controlling inflammation is key to managing symptoms and preventing joint damage.

MECHANISMS OF HORMONE ACTION

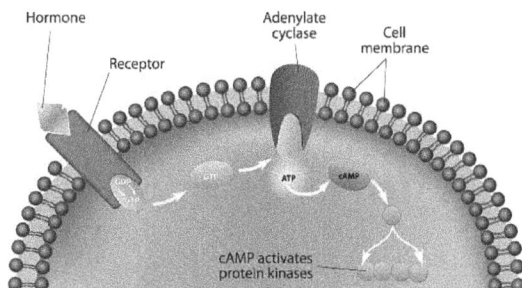

Hormone
Receptor
Adenylate cyclase
Cell membrane
ATP
cAMP
cAMP activates protein kinases

The potential of peptides extends into the realm of autoimmune diseases, where the immune system mistakenly attacks the body's own tissues. In conditions like rheumatoid arthritis, peptides offer a promising therapeutic approach by modulating immune activity to prevent unnecessary attacks on healthy cells. By restoring balance to the immune response, peptides can alleviate the symptoms of autoimmune diseases and improve quality of life. This modulation is akin to retraining the immune system, teaching it to distinguish between friend and foe. The precision of peptides in targeting specific pathways makes them ideal candidates for managing autoimmune conditions, where traditional treatments may fall short or cause unwanted side effects.

In addition to their regulatory roles, peptides are also pivotal in infection control. Antimicrobial peptides act as the body's natural antibiotics, directly targeting and destroying pathogens. These peptides can disrupt the membranes of bacteria, viruses, and fungi, rendering them harmless. This mechanism of action is crucial in an era where antibiotic resistance is a growing concern. By providing an alternative means of infection control, antimicrobial peptides help maintain the body's defenses against evolving threats. Their versatility and effectiveness make them a valuable asset in the ongoing battle against infectious diseases.

As we explore the role of peptides in inflammation and immunity, it becomes clear that they are indispensable allies in maintaining health. Their ability to modulate immune responses, control inflammation, and combat infections highlights their importance in both prevention and treatment. Peptides offer a targeted and nuanced approach to health optimization, addressing the complexities of the immune system with precision and efficacy. Their potential to enhance immune function, reduce inflammation, and manage autoimmune conditions elevates them as powerful tools in the pursuit of wellness. As we continue to uncover the myriad ways in which peptides influence our health, their promise as therapeutic agents become increasingly evident.

In the next chapter, we will delve into how peptides can be applied in real-world scenarios, from daily health routines to advanced therapeutic interventions. Through practical examples and case studies, we will see how the theoretical knowledge of peptide action translates into tangible health benefits.

Let's explore the exciting possibilities of integrating peptides into our lives for optimal health and vitality.

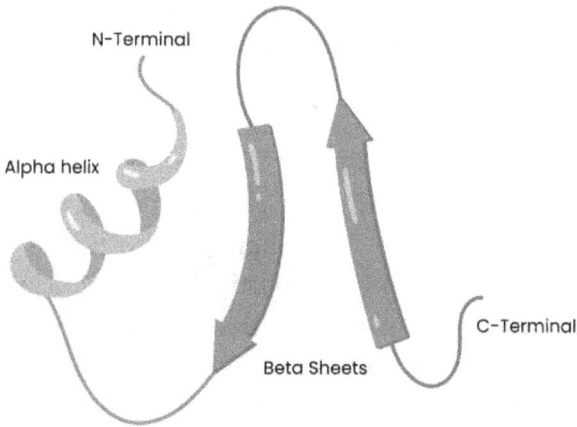

Chapter 3:
Peptides for Health and Longevity

In a quiet café, I once met Eleanor, a vibrant septuagenarian with a zest for life that belied her years. She leaned in, eyes sparkling, and asked me, "What if age really is just a number? Can we truly turn back the clock?" Her question resonated deeply, echoing the hopes and dreams of many who wish to age gracefully without losing vitality. This chapter delves into how peptides might hold the key to redefining aging, offering tools that could help maintain youthful energy and health.

As we explore the potential of anti-aging peptides, let's begin with Thymosin alpha-1 and Epithalon. Thymosin alpha-1 is a peptide naturally produced in the thymus gland, and it plays a vital role in immune function. It works by enhancing the body's ability to fight infections and diseases, a feature particularly beneficial as we age and our immune system weakens. Epithalon, on the other hand, is a peptide known for its potential to elongate telomeres, the protective caps on our chromosomes that shorten as we age. Telomeres act like the plastic tips on shoelaces, preventing genetic material from fraying. By preserving telomere length, Epithalon may help maintain cellular youthfulness and vitality, offering a promising avenue for those seeking to mitigate the effects of aging.

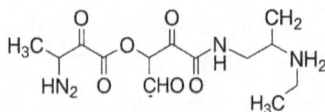

Epithalon

The mechanisms through which these peptides operate are as fascinating as they are complex. Thymosin alpha-1 works at the cellular level, enhancing immune responses by promoting the production of immune cells and modulating cytokine activity. This action not only bolsters the immune system but also aids in repairing DNA damage, a crucial factor in counteracting the aging process. Epithalon, meanwhile, stimulates the activity of telomerase, an enzyme that adds length to telomeres. This process helps delay the negative effects of cellular aging by allowing cells to divide healthily and efficiently. Additionally, these peptides stimulate antioxidant pathways, reducing oxidative stress—a major contributor to cellular aging. By mitigating the damage caused by free radicals, these peptides support the maintenance of cellular integrity and function.

Scientific research continues to shed light on the efficacy of these anti-aging peptides. Studies involving model organisms have shown that Thymosin alpha-1 can improve immune function, potentially extending lifespan by reducing the incidence of age-related diseases. Research has also demonstrated that Epithalon can increase the lifespan of certain organisms by maintaining telomere length and promoting overall cellular health. While human studies are still in progress, these findings offer hope for the development of peptide-based anti-aging therapies that could benefit us all. The scientific community is optimistic about the potential these peptides hold, and ongoing research aims to unlock their full capabilities.

For those interested in incorporating anti-aging peptides into their wellness routine, practical application and adherence to protocols are vital. Thymosin alpha-1 is typically administered via injection, with a recommended schedule of twice a week to maintain optimal immune function. Epithalon, often used in cycles, can be taken in various forms, including injections and oral supplements. Combining these peptides with other anti-aging interventions, such as a balanced diet and regular exercise, can enhance their effects. It's crucial to approach peptide use with caution and consultation from a healthcare provider to ensure safe and effective integration into your lifestyle.

For those eager to take control of their aging process, reflecting on your wellness goals and how these peptides align with your desired outcomes can be beneficial. Consider keeping a journal to track your experiences and any changes you notice in your energy levels, immune health, or overall well-being. This reflection can help you identify the benefits and make informed decisions about your health strategy.

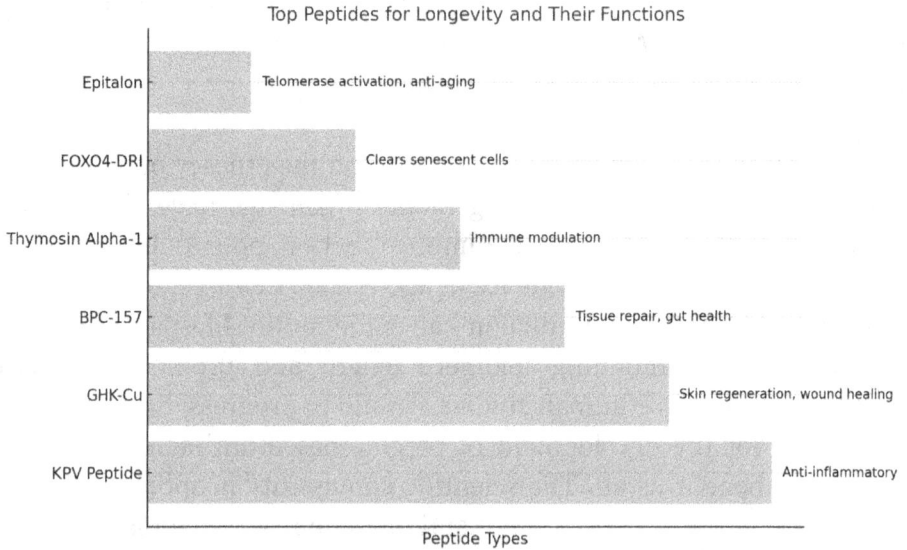

Top Peptides for Longevity and Their Functions

Peptide	Function
Epitalon	Telomerase activation, anti-aging
FOXO4-DRI	Clears senescent cells
Thymosin Alpha-1	Immune modulation
BPC-157	Tissue repair, gut health
GHK-Cu	Skin regeneration, wound healing
KPV Peptide	Anti-inflammatory

Peptide Types

Peptides for Fat Loss: Targeting Stubborn Areas

In the quest for weight management, many find themselves frustrated by stubborn fat that refuses to budge, despite rigorous exercise and a balanced diet. The potential of peptides offers a new frontier in addressing this challenge, providing tools that target fat reduction with precision. AOD9604 is one such peptide, designed specifically for targeted fat loss. Developed as a lipolytic fragment of human growth hormone, AOD9604 stimulates the breakdown of fat stores without affecting blood sugar or tissue growth. Its mechanism is straightforward yet effective. By activating lipolytic pathways, AOD9604 encourages the body to use stored fat as energy, making it a powerful ally in weight management.

Another notable peptide in the realm of weight management is Follistatin, which not only helps reduce fat but also preserves lean muscle mass. Follistatin works by inhibiting myostatin, a protein that limits muscle growth. This dual action makes it particularly appealing for those looking to sculpt their physique while shedding unwanted fat. By preserving muscle, Follistatin ensures that the metabolic rate remains high, facilitating further fat loss. This preservation is crucial, as muscle tissue burns more calories than fat, even at rest, making it a valuable component in any weight management strategy. The synergy of fat reduction and muscle preservation positions these peptides as versatile tools for achieving a leaner body.

The mechanisms driving fat loss with these peptides are rooted in their ability to disrupt the processes of fat storage and promote fat breakdown. AOD9604 inhibits lipogenesis, the creation of new fat cells, while simultaneously enhancing lipolysis, the process of breaking down existing fat cells. This dual approach ensures that not only is fat being used as energy, but the body is also less likely to store excess calories as fat. In this way, peptides align with the body's natural processes, encouraging a more efficient metabolism. The targeted nature of these actions allows for more precise management of body composition, addressing specific areas of concern and enhancing overall effectiveness.

Clinical trials have provided compelling evidence supporting the effectiveness of peptides in fat loss. Studies have shown that AOD9604, for example, can lead to significant changes in body composition, reducing body fat while maintaining lean muscle mass. These trials highlight the peptide's ability to enhance lipolytic sensitivity, thereby increasing the body's capacity to burn fat. The evidence is not just anecdotal; it is backed by rigorous scientific research that validates the potential of peptides as effective tools in weight management. Such findings bolster confidence in their use, providing a foundation for integrating peptides into a comprehensive wellness plan.

Incorporating peptides into a fat-loss program requires a multifaceted approach that includes lifestyle modifications. Combining peptide use with regular exercise and a balanced diet maximizes their effectiveness. Exercise, particularly strength training, complements the action of peptides by promoting muscle growth and enhancing metabolic rate. Meanwhile, a diet rich in whole foods supports the body's nutritional needs, ensuring that it operates optimally. Monitoring and adjusting peptide use based on individual response is crucial, as it allows for personalized optimization. Regular assessments of body composition and health markers can guide these adjustments, ensuring that the approach remains aligned with personal goals.

To aid in the effective use of peptides for fat loss, consider creating a checklist to track your progress and ensure adherence to your regimen. This checklist might include daily exercise, meal planning, and peptide administration, allowing you to visualize your commitment to your health goals. Such a tool can enhance motivation and accountability, serving as a practical companion in your weight management journey.

Enhancing Metabolism with Peptides: The Science Behind It

Imagine having a metabolism that runs like a finely-tuned engine, burning fuel efficiently and powering you through your day with energy to spare. Peptides, particularly CJC-1295 and Tesamorelin, offer intriguing possibilities for enhancing metabolic function, making this vision more attainable. CJC-1295, a growth hormone-releasing peptide, stimulates the release of growth hormone from the pituitary gland. This process not only promotes cell growth and regeneration but also boosts metabolic rate. By increasing growth hormone levels, CJC-1295 encourages your body to utilize energy more effectively, contributing to a more robust metabolism. Tesamorelin, on the other hand, is particularly noted for its ability to reduce abdominal fat. By mimicking growth hormone-releasing hormone (GHRH), Tesamorelin stimulates the natural release of growth hormone, enhancing metabolic processes and supporting fat reduction, particularly in the abdominal region. Both peptides work synergistically to optimize metabolic function, offering a promising approach to managing weight and enhancing overall energy levels.

At the core of these peptides' effectiveness is their interaction with metabolic pathways. They enhance mitochondrial function, which is crucial for energy production. Mitochondria, often referred to as the powerhouses of the cell, generates the energy necessary for cellular function. By boosting mitochondrial efficiency, these peptides ensure that your cells have the energy they need to perform at their best. This enhancement translates to increased energy expenditure, allowing your body to burn more calories even at rest. The upregulation of these pathways not only aids in weight management but also supports overall health by improving energy availability for vital bodily functions. This increased energy expenditure is particularly beneficial for those struggling with metabolic disorders like obesity and diabetes, where energy balance is often disrupted. By improving how your body processes and uses energy, these peptides offer a targeted approach to enhancing metabolic health.

HEALING WITH PEPTIDES: THE ULTIMATE GUIDE TO BIOHACKING YOUR BODY

HELP US GROW WITH YOUR REVIEW!

WE'D LOVE YOUR FEEDBACK!

THANK YOU FOR CHOOSING HEALING WITH PEPTIDES: THE ULTIMATE GUIDE TO BIOHACKING YOUR BODY AS PART OF YOUR HEALTH AND WELLNESS JOURNEY. YOUR FEEDBACK IS INCREDIBLY VALUABLE TO US! IF YOU FOUND THE INSIGHTS AND INFORMATION IN THIS BOOK HELPFUL, WE WOULD GREATLY APPRECIATE IT IF YOU COULD LEAVE A POSITIVE REVIEW. SIMPLY SCAN THE QR CODE BELOW TO SHARE YOUR THOUGHTS. YOUR REVIEW NOT ONLY SUPPORTS US IN REACHING MORE PEOPLE BUT ALSO HELPS TO SPREAD THE MESSAGE OF CUTTING-EDGE WELLNESS AND PEPTIDE-BASED HEALING.

THANK YOU FOR YOUR SUPPORT!

The potential benefits of peptides in managing metabolic disorders are significant. By enhancing insulin sensitivity, these peptides help your body respond more effectively to insulin, reducing the risk of insulin resistance—a precursor to type 2 diabetes. Improved insulin sensitivity means that your body can better regulate blood sugar levels, reducing the risk of spikes and crashes that can lead to energy slumps and cravings. This regulation is critical for maintaining steady energy levels and preventing the long-term complications associated with diabetes.

Additionally, by supporting fat reduction, especially in the abdominal area, these peptides help lower the risk of cardiovascular diseases often associated with obesity. The targeted nature of peptide action ensures that these benefits are achieved with precision, offering a promising solution for those seeking to manage their metabolic health more effectively.

Incorporating metabolism-enhancing peptides into your routine requires strategic planning. Timing and frequency of administration are crucial to maximizing their effects. Peptides like CJC-1295 and Tesamorelin are typically administered via injection, with protocols varying based on individual needs and goals. For optimal results, these peptides are often taken in cycles, with regular assessments to monitor progress and adjust dosages as needed.

This cyclical approach allows your body to adapt and respond effectively to the peptides, ensuring sustained benefits over time. Lifestyle modifications further enhance their impact. A balanced diet rich in whole foods provides the nutrients necessary for efficient energy production, while regular physical activity boosts metabolic rate and supports the effects of peptides. Combining these lifestyle changes with peptide therapy creates a holistic approach to metabolic health, empowering you to achieve and maintain a healthy weight and energy balance.

To effectively integrate these peptides into your wellness routine, consider setting realistic goals and tracking your progress. Keep a log of your energy levels, weight, and any changes in body composition. This practice not only helps you stay motivated but also provides valuable insights into how your body responds to the peptides. By understanding these changes, you can make informed decisions about your health strategy, adjusting as necessary to achieve your desired outcomes. Peptides offer a powerful tool for enhancing metabolism, but their success depends on a thoughtful and personalized approach.

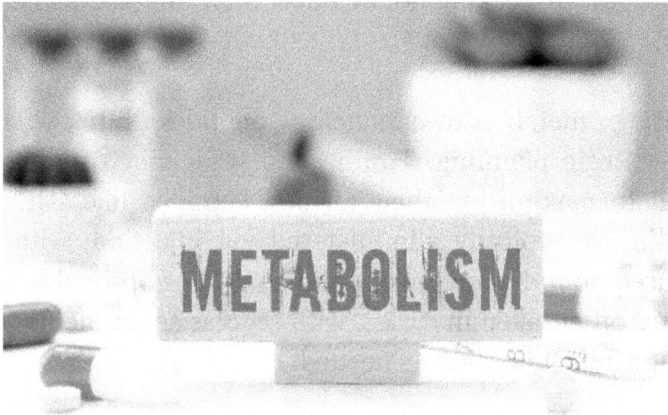

Peptides for Bone and Joint Health: Strengthening from Within

Picture your skeletal system as the backbone of not just your body, but your daily life, enabling everything from a simple walk in the park to a vigorous workout at the gym. It's easy to take for granted until you feel an ache in your knee or a twinge in your back. This is where peptides like BPC-157 and MK-677 come into play, offering promising solutions to support and enhance bone and joint health. BPC-157, a peptide derived from a protein found in the stomach, has gained attention for its remarkable ability to aid in joint repair. It targets the healing process directly, accelerating recovery from injuries by promoting blood vessel growth and collagen production. This is particularly beneficial for those with joint issues, as collagen is a key structural component of ligaments and tendons, providing the strength and flexibility needed for mobility.

Meanwhile, MK-677, known for its growth hormone secretagogue properties, shines in the realm of bone health by improving bone density. By stimulating the secretion of growth hormones, MK-677 enhances osteoblast activity—cells responsible for bone formation. This action not only strengthens existing bones but also contributes to the development of new bone tissue, crucial for maintaining skeletal integrity as we age. The enhancement of bone density can significantly reduce the risk of fractures, a common concern, especially among the elderly. These peptides work in synergy, with BPC-157 focusing on joint repair and MK-677 on bone strengthening, together providing a comprehensive approach to skeletal health.

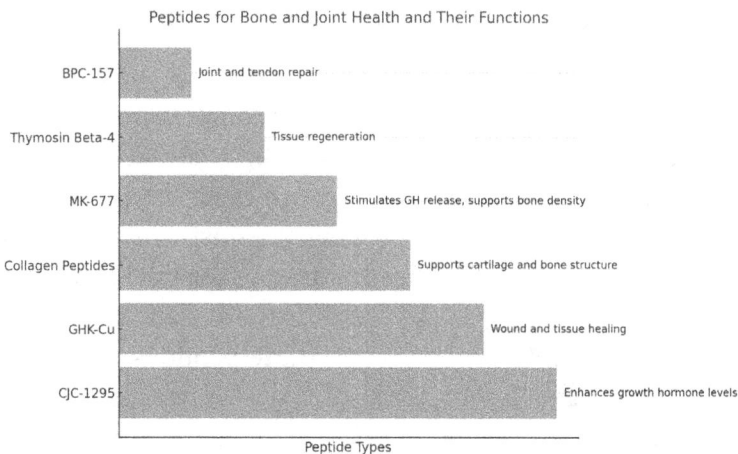

Peptides for Bone and Joint Health and Their Functions

Peptide Types	
BPC-157	Joint and tendon repair
Thymosin Beta-4	Tissue regeneration
MK-677	Stimulates GH release, supports bone density
Collagen Peptides	Supports cartilage and bone structure
GHK-Cu	Wound and tissue healing
CJC-1295	Enhances growth hormone levels

The systems behind these peptides are supported by compelling research. Studies have demonstrated BPC-157's efficacy in accelerating the healing of tendon and ligament injuries, reducing recovery time, and improving overall joint function. In experimental models, BPC-157 has been shown to enhance the healing of muscle tears and promote vascularization, ensuring that nutrients and oxygen are efficiently delivered to damaged tissues. Similarly, MK-677 has been studied for its effects on bone metabolism, with findings indicating significant improvements in bone density. Research involving MK-677 has shown increased markers of bone formation, suggesting its potential in treating conditions like osteoporosis. These studies provide a solid foundation for using peptides in maintaining and enhancing bone and joint health, offering a scientific basis for their application.

For those considering peptide use to support joint health, it's important to approach it with a well-rounded strategy. Integrating these peptides into a joint health regimen can be particularly beneficial for athletes, the elderly, or anyone recovering from joint injuries. For BPC-157, protocols typically involve consistent administration to maximize its healing benefits. It's often most effective when used in conjunction with physical therapy, which can help restore joint function and prevent future injuries. Physical therapy exercises complement the peptide's action, reinforcing the healing process and strengthening the surrounding muscles and tissues.

Similarly, MK-677's effects on bone density can be part of a broader strategy that includes weight-bearing exercises and a diet rich in calcium and vitamin D. These lifestyle components work alongside MK-677 to optimize bone health, ensuring that bones remain strong and resilient. Regular monitoring through bone density scans can help track progress and make any necessary adjustments to the regimen. For individuals looking to improve their skeletal health, combining these peptides with lifestyle changes offers a holistic approach that can lead to lasting benefits. As you incorporate peptides into your routine, keep in mind the importance of consistency and patience, as improvements in bone and joint health can take time to manifest.

Skin Health and Peptides: A Youthful Glow

Imagine the skin as the canvas of our body, reflecting not just age but health and vitality. As time progresses, maintaining that youthful glow often becomes a challenge due to environmental stressors and the natural aging process. This is where the transformative potential of peptides like Matrixyl and GHK-Cu comes into play. Matrixyl, a peptide renowned for its ability to boost collagen production, acts like a master artist, filling in the fine lines and wrinkles that gradually appear over time. Collagen, a structural protein, provides the skin with firmness and elasticity, and its production naturally declines with age. By stimulating collagen synthesis,

Matrixyl helps restore the skin's youthful resilience, offering a non-invasive alternative to cosmetic procedures. Meanwhile, GHK-Cu, a copper peptide, stands out for its remarkable wound healing and skin remodeling capabilities. This peptide, likened to a skilled restorer, not only accelerates the healing of damaged tissue but also enhances the skin's overall appearance by promoting a more even tone and texture. GHK-Cu's role in skin health is crucial, as it assists in cellular communication, promoting the migration of repair cells to sites of damage and encouraging new cell growth, which is essential for skin renewal.

The mechanisms behind skin rejuvenation with these peptides are both intriguing and effective. At the cellular level, peptides promote fibroblast activity, which is vital for maintaining skin structure. Fibroblasts, the cells responsible for producing collagen and other extracellular matrix components, are stimulated by these peptides to enhance their activity. Additionally, peptides help reduce oxidative stress in skin cells, a process that combats the damage caused by free radicals. These unstable molecules contribute to the aging process by breaking down collagen and elastin, leading to sagging skin and wrinkles. By neutralizing free radicals, peptides protect the skin from premature aging and environmental damage, contributing to a healthier complexion.

Scientific research supports the benefits of peptides in skin health. Clinical trials have demonstrated that peptides like Matrixyl can significantly reduce the appearance of fine lines and wrinkles, providing a visible lift to aging skin. In one study, participants using a peptide-based cream showed a marked improvement in skin texture and elasticity after just a few weeks. Similarly, GHK-Cu has been extensively studied for its wound-healing properties, with results indicating faster healing times and improved skin clarity. These findings underscore the potential of peptides as effective tools for skin rejuvenation, offering a scientific foundation for their use in skincare regimens.

Incorporating peptides into a skincare routine involves strategic application techniques to maximize their benefits. Topical formulations, such as creams and serums, are the most common methods of delivery, allowing peptides to penetrate the skin and exert their effects. For optimal results, it's important to apply these products to clean skin, ideally after cleansing and before moisturizing, to ensure maximum absorption. Combining peptides with other skincare agents, such as antioxidants or hyaluronic acid, can enhance their efficacy. Antioxidants work synergistically with peptides to provide an additional layer of protection against environmental damage, while hyaluronic acid helps retain skin moisture, further plumping and smoothing the complexion.

For those eager to see how peptides can transform their skin, consider setting up a simple experiment at home. Choose a peptide-based product and apply it consistently for several weeks, monitoring changes in skin texture, firmness, and overall appearance. Keep a journal to note any improvements or changes and take before-and-after photos to visually track progress. This practice not only helps you assess the effectiveness of peptides in your skincare routine but also encourages a personalized approach to skin health, allowing you to adapt and refine your regimen based on observed results.

The Role of Peptides in Cardiovascular Health

As we explore the realm of cardiovascular health, the significance of peptides becomes increasingly apparent. The heart and vascular system require constant support to function optimally, and peptides like angiotensin-converting enzyme (ACE) inhibitors and BPC-157 offer promising avenues to achieve this. ACE inhibitors are well-known for their role in regulating blood pressure, acting by preventing the conversion of angiotensin I to angiotensin II, a potent vasoconstrictor. This process helps relax blood vessels, ultimately reducing blood pressure and alleviating the strain on your heart. By moderating blood pressure, ACE inhibitors can significantly decrease the risk of heart-related complications, providing a protective shield for your cardiovascular system.

On the other hand, BPC-157, a peptide derived from a portion of a gastric juice protein, shows potential in supporting vascular repair. This peptide enhances the healing of blood vessels, especially after injury or stress, by promoting angiogenesis, the formation of new blood vessels. This ability to stimulate vascular repair makes BPC-157 a valuable tool in addressing cardiovascular issues, as it aids in maintaining the integrity and function of blood vessels. Furthermore, BPC-157 exhibits anti-inflammatory properties, reducing inflammation in cardiovascular tissues and supporting overall heart health. By mitigating inflammation, this peptide helps prevent the progression of cardiovascular diseases, offering another layer of protection for your heart and blood vessels.

The mechanisms by which these peptides support cardiovascular health are well-documented in scientific studies. Research indicates that ACE inhibitors not only lower blood pressure but also improve cardiac output, the amount of blood the heart pumps with each beat. This enhancement in cardiac function can lead to better oxygen delivery throughout the body, improving overall vitality.

Studies also show that ACE inhibitors can reduce arterial plaque formation, decreasing the risk of atherosclerosis—a condition characterized by the buildup of fatty deposits in the arteries that can lead to heart attacks and strokes. These findings underscore the importance of peptides in maintaining cardiovascular health and preventing disease.

BPC-157's impact on heart health is equally impressive. Research demonstrates its ability to reduce oxidative stress in the cardiovascular system, protecting heart tissue from damage caused by free radicals. By promoting the repair and regeneration of blood vessels, BPC-157 supports healthy circulation, ensuring that nutrients and oxygen are efficiently delivered to tissues. This peptide's role in vascular health extends to its potential use in treating conditions such as hypertension and heart failure, where improved blood flow and reduced inflammation are crucial for recovery. The evidence supporting BPC-157's cardiovascular benefits highlights its potential as a therapeutic option for those seeking to enhance heart health and prevent disease.

When considering the integration of peptides into a cardiovascular health regimen, it's important to follow practical protocols. For ACE inhibitors, dosing should be personalized based on individual needs and monitored by a healthcare professional to ensure optimal blood pressure control without adverse effects. Combining these peptides with lifestyle interventions can further enhance their benefits. A heart-healthy diet rich in fruits, vegetables, whole grains, and lean proteins supports cardiovascular function by providing essential nutrients and antioxidants.

Regular physical activity, such as brisk walking or cycling, strengthens the heart muscle and improves circulation, complementing the effects of peptides. By adopting these lifestyle changes in conjunction with the use of peptide, you can create a comprehensive approach to cardiovascular health that maximizes benefits and minimizes risks.

To further personalize your approach to cardiovascular health, consider keeping a journal to track your blood pressure, heart rate, and overall well-being. This practice allows you to monitor changes over time and make informed decisions about your health strategy. By understanding how your body responds to peptides and lifestyle modifications, you can tailor your regimen to better meet your needs and goals. Peptides offer a powerful tool for supporting cardiovascular health, but their success depends on thoughtful integration into a holistic wellness plan.

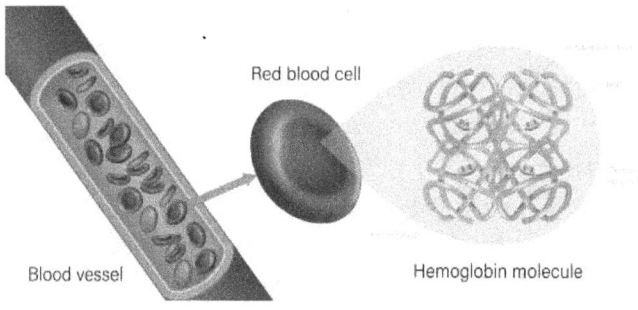

Red blood cell

Blood vessel

Hemoglobin molecule

Chapter 4:
Personalized Peptide Protocols

In the world of health optimization, one size rarely fits all. Each of us is a unique tapestry of experiences, challenges, and aspirations, and our approach to wellness should reflect this individuality. Consider the story of Tom, a middle-aged professional who found himself at a crossroads. Despite regular exercise and a balanced diet, he struggled with persistent fatigue and a lack of focus. As we explored his goals, it became clear that a tailored peptide plan could be the key to unlocking his potential. This chapter is about crafting your own personalized peptide protocol, a roadmap designed to align with your specific health objectives and lifestyle.

The first step in creating your peptide plan is to define your health goals clearly. What do you hope to achieve? Whether it's muscle gain, fat loss, anti-aging, or improved mental clarity, setting specific targets will guide your peptide choices. If anti-aging is your focus, peptides known for supporting cellular repair and vitality are the best choice. Improved mental clarity might involve peptides that enhance neurotransmitter function. By clearly identifying these goals, you set the foundation for a targeted and effective peptide regimen.

Next, assess your personal health status and needs. This involves taking stock of your current health conditions, lifestyle, and any existing medical concerns. Consideration of these factors is crucial, as they influence how your body responds to peptides. For instance, if you have a history of joint issues, peptides that support connective tissue health could be prioritized. Baseline measurements, such as body composition or blood markers, provide a starting point for your journey.

These metrics help tailor your peptide use, ensuring it aligns with your unique physiology and health status. It's a bit like plotting a course on a map; you need to know your starting point to plan the best route to your destination.

Once you've defined your goals and assessed your health, it's time to determine realistic outcomes and timelines. Setting achievable expectations is key to maintaining motivation and tracking progress. Short-term goals might focus on immediate benefits, such as increased energy or improved sleep, while long-term goals could encompass more significant changes, like sustained weight loss or enhanced cognitive function. Establishing milestones along the way provides checkpoints to celebrate progress and make necessary adjustments. This approach mirrors the concept of a marathon rather than a sprint, emphasizing sustainable change over quick fixes.

With your objectives, health status, and timelines in place, you can develop a customized peptide roadmap. This involves selecting specific peptides that align with your goals and integrating them into your daily routine. For muscle gain, peptides like CJC-1295 with Ipamorelin might be considered, as they enhance growth hormone release and muscle recovery (Source 1). For those targeting fat loss, AOD9604 is known for its ability to promote fat breakdown without affecting muscle mass (Source 2). The key is to choose peptides that complement your goals and fit seamlessly into your lifestyle. Incorporating peptides into your routine can be as simple as scheduling them alongside meals or workouts, ensuring consistency and adherence.

To support your journey, consider keeping a health journal to track your experiences and progress. This can include noting changes in energy levels, mood, and physical performance, as well as any challenges you encounter. By documenting your journey, you create a valuable resource for reflection and adjustment, allowing you to refine your approach as needed. This practice not only enhances self-awareness but also empowers you to take an active role in your health journey, ensuring that your peptide plan remains a dynamic and evolving tool for wellness.

Dosage and Cycling: Mastering the Art of Peptide Use

Understanding the proper dosage for peptides is crucial. It's the difference between achieving desired effects and experiencing unwanted side effects. Proper dosing begins with guidelines tailored to each peptide and user. For example, starting doses for peptides such as CJC-1295 with DAC are typically around 1-2 mg once or twice weekly, while BPC-157 is often recommended at 200 mcg to 500 mcg daily. These starting points provide a baseline, allowing you to observe how your body reacts before making any adjustments.

Adjustments are a fundamental part of the process as you take into account your personal responses. This could mean increasing or decreasing the dose based on factors like effectiveness and any side effects you might experience. It's important to approach dosage with flexibility, recognizing that what works for one person may not work for another. Consulting with a healthcare professional before making any changes is always advisable to ensure safety and efficacy.

Cycling peptides can significantly enhance their effectiveness while minimizing potential downsides. The concept of cycling involves alternating between periods of peptide use (on-cycle) and periods of rest (off-cycle). This strategy prevents the body from becoming too accustomed to the peptide, maintaining its responsiveness over time. On-cycle periods might last anywhere from 8 to 12 weeks, followed by an off-cycle period of 4 to 6 weeks.

This break allows your body to reset, reducing the likelihood of desensitization or diminishing returns. The frequency and duration of cycles should align with individual goals and the specific peptides in use. For instance, growth hormone-releasing peptides might have different cycle lengths compared to those used primarily for fat loss or muscle repair. By incorporating cycling into your regimen, you maximize the long-term benefits of peptides, ensuring that they remain an effective tool in your health optimization toolkit.

Providing general dosing protocols offers a framework adaptable to individual needs. For peptides like Ipamorelin, dosing might range from 200 mcg to 300 mcg per day, divided into two doses. This flexibility allows you to find the sweet spot that aligns with your body's unique requirements. Over time, as you become more attuned to your body's responses, you can adjust doses as needed. This might involve gradually increasing doses to enhance effects or reducing them if side effects occur. Monitoring your body's reactions is key, as it provides the insights needed to tailor your peptide use effectively.

Remember, peptides are not a one-size-fits-all solution. They require personalization to unlock their full potential, and being open to adjustments is part of that process.

Several factors influence the appropriate dosage of peptides, including age, weight, and overall health status. Age can affect how your body metabolizes peptides, with younger individuals typically having a faster metabolism compared to older adults. This variability may necessitate different dosing strategies, ensuring that each person receives the optimal amount for their needs. Weight also plays a role, as it affects how substances are distributed throughout the body. Heavier individuals might require higher doses to achieve similar effects as someone with a lower body weight.

Additionally, underlying health conditions can impact how peptides are processed and should be considered when determining dosages. For example, a person with metabolic issues might need to approach dosing differently than someone without such concerns. Lifestyle factors, such as activity level and diet, further influence how your body responds to peptides, making it crucial to consider these elements when crafting your peptide protocol.

Visual Element: Dosage and Cycling Checklist

- Starting Dose: **Begin with the lowest recommended dose for your chosen peptide.**
- Adjustment Phase: **Monitor response for 2-4 weeks; adjust dose based on effectiveness and side effects.**
- Cycling: **Implement on-cycle (8-12 weeks) and off-cycle (4-6 weeks) periods.**
- Individual Factors: **Consider age, weight, and health status to tailor dosing.**
- Consultation: **Regular check-ins with a healthcare provider to ensure safety and effectiveness.**

Peptide Stacking: Creating Synergistic Effects

Think of peptide stacking like crafting a masterful recipe, where each ingredient enhances the other to create a dish that's greater than the sum of its parts. By combining multiple peptides, you can amplify their benefits, achieving results that are more pronounced and tailored to your specific health goals. This concept of synergy means that when peptides are stacked together, they can work in tandem to enhance each other, providing a more comprehensive approach to health optimization. For instance, when targeting muscle growth, stacking peptides like CJC-1295 with Ipamorelin can significantly boost growth hormone levels, improve protein synthesis, and enhance recovery. This combination not only supports muscle gain but also aids in fat burning, making it a powerful stack for those looking to improve body composition (Source 1).

Selecting the right peptides to stack involves understanding how they interact and complement each other. For cognitive enhancement, pairing peptides that support neurotransmitter function with those that promote neuroprotection can create a robust protocol for mental clarity and focus. For example, combining peptides like Selank, which reduces anxiety and enhances cognitive function, with Cerebrolysin, known for its neuroprotective properties, can result in improved mental performance and resilience. This approach allows you to customize your stack based on the specific cognitive challenges you face and the specific results you desire, whether it's improving focus, boosting memory, or reducing stress-related cognitive decline.

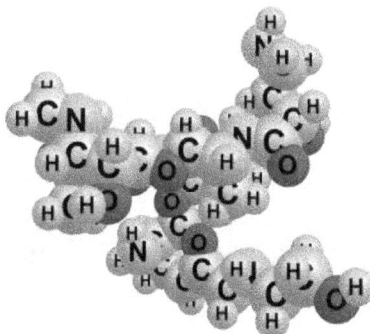

While the benefits of stacking peptides are enticing, it's crucial to consider the potential risks involved. The increased efficacy from stacking can also lead to amplified side effects if not carefully monitored. It's important to pay attention to how your body responds to each stack, as individual reactions can vary. Some may experience enhanced benefits with minimal side effects, while others may need to adjust doses or switch peptides to avoid adverse reactions. Regular monitoring, possibly through health journals or apps, can help track these responses, allowing for timely adjustments to your regimen. Consulting with a healthcare professional familiar with peptide use can offer valuable insights and guidance, ensuring your stacks are both effective and safe.

To illustrate the potential of peptide stacking, let's explore some example protocols. For athletic performance, one might consider a stack that includes CJC-1295 with Ipamorelin for muscle growth and recovery, BPC-157 for reducing inflammation and supporting joint health, and TB-500 for additional healing and flexibility benefits. This stack not only targets muscle growth but also addresses recovery and injury prevention, creating a well-rounded approach to athletic enhancement. For anti-aging purposes, a stack could include peptides like Epithalon, known for its telomere-supporting properties, combined with Thymosin alpha-1 for immune system support and GHK-Cu for skin rejuvenation. This combination targets multiple aspects of aging, from cellular health and immune function to skin vitality, offering a comprehensive anti-aging strategy.

The art of peptide stacking lies in the thoughtful selection and combination of peptides that align with your goals, taking into account your body's unique response to each one. This customization ensures that your peptide regimen is as effective as possible, maximizing benefits while minimizing risks. By understanding the principles of synergy and being mindful of potential side effects, you can create a peptide stack that unlocks new levels of health and performance, tailored to your individual needs and aspirations.

Age-Specific Peptide Protocols: Young Adults to Seniors

As we navigate through the different stages of life, our health priorities and physiological needs evolve and change, requiring tailored approaches to wellness. Peptides, with their diverse applications, offer strategic benefits that align with these changing needs. For young adults, the focus often shifts towards enhancing physical performance and building resilience against the pressures of modern life. Peptides that boost endurance, muscle recovery, and energy levels can be particularly valuable. Consider peptides like Ipamorelin and CJC-1295, which support growth hormone release, aiding in muscle repair and fat metabolism. These peptides can help young adults maximize their physical potential, whether it's excelling in sports or maintaining fitness amidst a busy schedule. Their ability to lessen recovery times and increase energy levels ensures that young adults can maintain a high level of activity without succumbing to burnout or injury, providing a solid foundation for a lifetime of health and vitality.

For seniors, the emphasis often shifts towards maintaining vitality and longevity. As the body ages, natural processes like collagen production and cellular regeneration slow down, leading to issues such as joint pain and reduced energy levels. Peptides can help mitigate these effects by promoting cellular repair and supporting joint health. BPC-157 is a popular choice for seniors due to its ability to enhance healing and reduce inflammation, offering relief from joint discomfort and supporting an active lifestyle. Similarly, Thymosin alpha-1 can boost immune function, a critical concern for older adults whose immune responses may weaken over time. By incorporating peptides that support these functions, seniors can enhance their quality of life, staying active and engaged in their pursuits. These peptides not only target physical health but also contribute to mental clarity and emotional well-being, allowing seniors to enjoy their golden years with vigor and enthusiasm.

The physiological differences between age groups significantly influence the effectiveness and safety of peptide use. Younger individuals often have faster metabolisms, which can impact how quickly peptides are absorbed and utilized by the body. This rapid absorption can enhance the effectiveness of peptides aimed at muscle growth and recovery, making them particularly beneficial for young adults who engage in rigorous physical activities. In contrast, seniors may experience slower metabolic rates, which can affect how peptides are processed and necessitate adjustments in dosing to achieve optimal outcomes. Age-related health concerns, such as cardiovascular issues or hormonal imbalances, also play a role in peptide selection, as these factors can influence both the efficacy and safety of peptide therapies. Understanding these differences is crucial for designing age-appropriate peptide protocols that maximize benefits while minimizing risks.

Designing age-specific peptide plans involves crafting structured protocols that cater to the distinct needs of each age group. For those in middle age, enhancing youthfulness and vitality often becomes a priority. Peptides that support skin health, such as GHK-Cu, can promote collagen production and improve skin elasticity, combating the visible signs of aging. These peptides, when combined with a healthy lifestyle, can help maintain a youthful appearance and vitality, providing a boost to confidence and well-being during this pivotal life stage. For seniors, protocols may focus on supporting joint health and cognitive function, addressing common concerns such as arthritis and memory decline.

Peptides like TB-500 can aid in reducing joint inflammation and promoting tissue repair, while those that support neuroprotection can help maintain cognitive clarity and enhance mental acuity. By tailoring peptide plans to address these specific concerns, individuals can effectively manage age-related challenges and enjoy a higher quality of life.

Age-related goals vary across demographics, reflecting the diverse priorities and challenges faced at each stage of life. For adults in the prime of their careers, managing stress and maintaining mental clarity are often top concerns. Peptides that support neurotransmitter balance and reduce stress can provide valuable support, enhancing focus and productivity in demanding environments. These peptides, when integrated into a comprehensive wellness plan, can help adults navigate the complexities of modern life with resilience and composure. In contrast, aging populations may prioritize cognitive support and physical vitality, seeking to preserve their independence and mental sharpness. Peptides that enhance brain health and support muscle maintenance can play a pivotal role in achieving these objectives, allowing seniors to remain active and engaged in their communities. By recognizing and addressing these age-specific goals, individuals can harness the power of peptides to support their unique health journeys, ensuring that each stage of life is lived to its fullest potential.

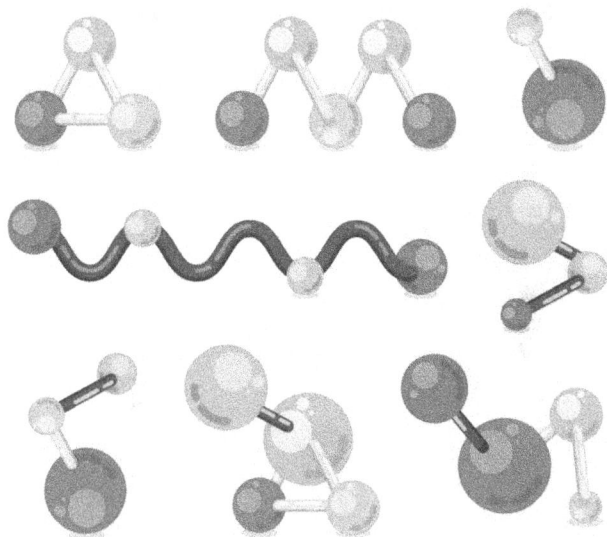

° MOLECULES COLLECTION °

Managing Side Effects: Ensuring Safe Peptide Use

Navigating the world of peptides can be rewarding, but it's important to remain vigilant about potential side effects. Understanding these effects is crucial to ensuring a safe and beneficial experience. Common side effects include injection site reactions, such as redness, swelling, or mild irritation. These are typically short-lived and resolve on their own. However, if you notice persistent discomfort, it might be wise to reassess your injection technique. Another potential issue is hormonal imbalances. Peptides that influence hormone levels might cause fluctuations, leading to symptoms like fatigue, mood changes, or even sleep disturbances. Recognizing these signs early allows you to make necessary adjustments before more significant issues arise.

To minimize risks, adopting best practices is essential. Proper injection techniques can significantly reduce the likelihood of adverse reactions. Always use sterile equipment and ensure the injection site is clean to prevent infections. Rotating injection sites is another practical tip. This helps prevent irritation and allows the skin to heal. Gradual dose escalation is another strategy; starting with a lower dose can help your body adjust gradually and reduce the risk of side effects. This approach is particularly beneficial for those new to peptides, as it allows you to monitor how your body responds without overwhelming your system. By introducing peptides slowly, you give yourself the chance to identify any potential adverse reactions early on.

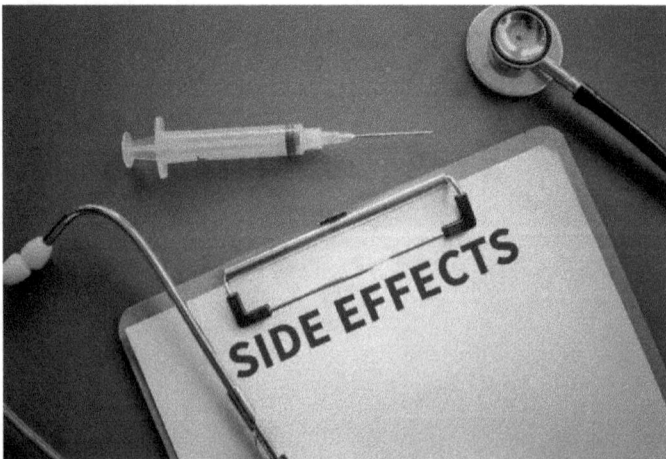

When side effects do occur, knowing how to respond is key. If you experience mild side effects, reducing the dose can often provide relief. For more persistent issues, discontinuing use temporarily might be necessary. It's always a good idea to consult with a healthcare professional if you're unsure about how to proceed. They can offer guidance tailored to your specific situation, ensuring that your peptide use is both safe and effective. Consulting a professional is particularly important if you experience more severe reactions, as it may indicate an underlying issue that needs addressing. Having a plan in place for dealing with side effects can provide peace of mind, allowing you to focus on the benefits that peptides can offer.

Maintaining safe practices for peptide administration is non-negotiable. Sterile handling and storage are fundamental to prevent contamination and ensure the efficacy of your peptides. Store them in a refrigerator, as this helps preserve their stability and potency. Monitoring for allergic reactions is another critical aspect. While rare, allergic reactions can occur, manifesting as hives, difficulty breathing, or swelling. If you notice any of these symptoms, seek medical attention immediately. Regularly reviewing your administration practices can help maintain safety and efficacy, ensuring that your peptides continue to support your health goals without unnecessary risk. By prioritizing safety, you build a solid foundation for successful peptide use.

In addition to these practices, consider setting up a system for regular self-assessment. This might include keeping a journal to track your experiences and noting any changes in how you feel. By consistently monitoring your body's responses, you gain valuable insights into what works for you and what doesn't. This proactive approach allows you to make informed decisions about your peptide use, optimizing your regimen for maximum benefit. Over time, you'll become more attuned to your body's signals, empowering you to manage side effects effectively and confidently.

Monitoring and Adjusting: How to Track Your Peptide Progress

Embracing peptide therapy is not just about selecting the right peptides and dosages; it's about continuously monitoring and adjusting your approach to ensure optimal results. Tracking your progress plays a pivotal role in this process. Imagine tracking as the compass guiding you toward your health goals, ensuring you're on the right path and making the necessary course corrections as needed. Utilizing health journals or tracking apps can be invaluable tools in this endeavor. These resources allow you to document your experiences, noting changes in your physical and mental well-being. By consistently recording data, you create a tangible record of your journey, making it easier to identify patterns and assess the efficacy of your peptide regimen.

Setting up a system for regular assessments is another cornerstone of successful peptide use. Regular health check-ins and tests provide crucial insights into your body's response to the peptides. These assessments might include routine blood tests, hormone panels, or body composition analyses, all of which offer a clearer picture of how your body is adapting. Comparing these results against your initial baseline measurements helps you gauge progress and determine if adjustments are necessary. These comparisons act as checkpoints, allowing you to celebrate successes and identify areas needing attention. Establishing a routine for these assessments ensures that you remain proactive, rather than reactive, in managing your health.

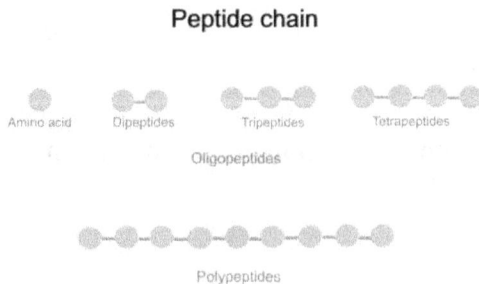

Peptide chain

Amino acid   Dipeptides   Tripeptides   Tetrapeptides

Oligopeptides

Polypeptides

The ability to make informed adjustments based on feedback is critical in optimizing your peptide protocol. As you track your progress, you may find that certain aspects of your regimen require tweaking. This might involve increasing or decreasing your dosage to better align with your body's needs or adding or removing specific peptides based on your current health objectives. The key is to remain flexible and open to change, recognizing that your body's needs can evolve. By being attentive to the feedback your body provides, you can refine your approach, ensuring that your peptide use continues to support your overarching health goals.

Using data to optimize peptide use involves leveraging the information you've gathered to make strategic decisions. This process resembles a feedback loop, where continuous improvement and adaptation are central to success. Analyzing the data collected through your tracking efforts helps you gain valuable insights into what works best for your body. These insights empower you to tailor your strategies, enhancing the effectiveness of your peptide regimen. The ability to adapt and respond to changes ensures that your approach remains dynamic, capable of evolving alongside your health journey.

Incorporating a regular review of your data can help maintain focus and motivation. Set aside time each month to evaluate your progress, reflecting on how your regimen is impacting your health. This practice not only reinforces accountability but also fosters a deeper understanding of your body's unique responses. By continually seeking improvement, you cultivate a mindset of growth and adaptability, qualities that are essential in achieving long-term health and wellness.

Peptide therapy, when monitored and adjusted effectively, can be a powerful tool in your health arsenal. As you refine your approach, keep in mind the broader context of your wellness goals, ensuring that each adjustment aligns with your vision for health. In the next chapter, we'll explore the real-world applications and success stories of peptides, offering practical insights into how these powerful molecules are transforming lives.

Chapter 5:
Real World Applications and Success Stories

Imagine standing in front of your bathroom mirror, scrutinizing the fine lines that have slowly crept onto your face over the years. This was the daily ritual for Margaret, a 62-year-old retiree who had always taken pride in her youthful appearance. Despite her best efforts with creams and serums, she noticed her skin losing its elasticity and her vitality waning. Her energy levels were not what they used to be, often leaving her fatigued by midday. The thought of aging gracefully seemed increasingly distant, and she longed for a solution that could restore her vigor.

Margaret's journey with anti-aging peptides began with a desire to reclaim her youthful glow and regain her energy. Her primary concerns revolved around the loss of skin elasticity and the decline in her stamina. After consulting with a health specialist, she decided to explore peptide therapy, focusing on two peptides renowned for their rejuvenating properties: Epithalon and GHK-Cu. The choice was not random; these peptides were selected for their targeted benefits. Epithalon, known for its ability to support telomere health, offered hope for slowing down the cellular aging process. Promoting the maintenance of telomerest helps cells function optimally for a longer period. Meanwhile, GHK-Cu, a peptide with copper-binding properties, was chosen for its remarkable effects on skin health. GHK-Cu has been shown to improve skin firmness and elasticity by stimulating collagen production and aiding in the repair of damaged tissues (Source 1). This dual approach aimed to address both skin and energy concerns.

As Margaret embarked on her peptide regimen, she began to notice subtle yet significant changes. Within weeks, her skin appeared more radiant and firmer, as if the clock had turned back. The fine lines that once traced her smile softened, and her complexion brightened. This transformation was not just skin-deep; she felt a newfound energy coursing through her veins. Tasks that once left her drained became manageable, and her afternoons were no longer plagued by fatigue. Quantitatively, her dermatologist noted a marked improvement in skin elasticity, confirming the visual changes Margaret observed. Qualitatively, her emotional well-being soared. The boost in vitality and appearance revitalized her confidence, lifting her spirits and enhancing her outlook on life.

Margaret's experience with anti-aging peptides underscored several valuable lessons. The synergy between Epithalon and GHK-Cu not only rejuvenated her skin but also reinvigorated her energy levels, illustrating the holistic benefits of peptide therapy. Her success prompted a deeper exploration into the potential of peptides, considering expanding their use for other aspects of health optimization. This experience led her to integrate peptide therapy into a broader anti-aging strategy, combining it with a balanced diet, regular exercise, and mindfulness practices. By adopting a comprehensive approach to wellness, Margaret ensured that the benefits of peptides were sustained and complemented by other healthy habits.

Reflection Section: Your Anti-Aging Checklist

- Identify Your Goals: **What are your primary concerns about aging? Consider both physical and emotional aspects.**
- Consult with a Professional: **Discuss potential peptide options with a healthcare provider to tailor a regimen to your personal needs.**
- Monitor Your Progress: **Keep a journal to track changes in skin appearance and energy levels. Note any improvements or side effects.**
- Adopt a Holistic Approach: **Combine peptide therapy with lifestyle changes such as nutrition, exercise, and stress management.**
- Reassess and Adjust: **Periodically evaluate your regimen's effectiveness and make necessary adjustments with your provider's guidance.**

Margaret's story is a testament to the transformative power of peptides in the pursuit of aging gracefully. Her journey highlights the potential of peptide therapy to rejuvenate not only the body but also the spirit, offering a glimpse into the possibilities of enhanced vitality and well-being.

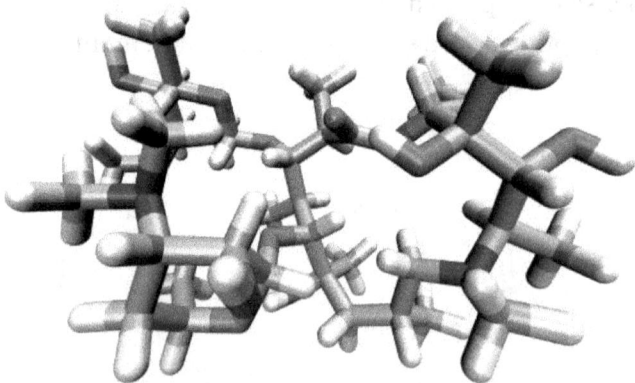

Overcoming Plateaus: A Fitness Journey with Peptides

Imagine standing in front of the mirror, flexing muscles that no longer seem to grow despite hours spent at the gym. This was the reality for Alex, a dedicated athlete who found himself stuck in a frustrating plateau. Despite his rigorous training routine, his muscle growth had stagnated, and the gains he once celebrated seemed like distant memories. Alex's frustration was palpable. He felt he was pouring effort into a bottomless well with no tangible returns. The weights felt heavier, the reps felt longer, and his motivation was waning. It was a classic case of hitting a wall, and Alex needed a strategy to break through.

In search of a solution, Alex turned to peptides, specifically Growth Hormone Releasing Peptides (GHRP) and Ipamorelin. The choice of GHRP was strategic. These peptides stimulate the pituitary gland to release growth hormone, an essential player in muscle development and repair. By increasing growth hormone levels, Alex aimed to reignite his muscle-building potential, expecting this would help him push past the stagnation. Meanwhile, Ipamorelin was chosen for its powerful effects on recovery.

Unlike other growth hormone secretagogues, Ipamorelin has a unique ability to enhance recovery without the unwanted side effects of increased appetite or cortisol release. This dual approach was designed to not only boost muscle gain but also improve recovery times, allowing Alex to train harder and more effectively.

With the peptide regimen underway, changes came swiftly. Alex noticed a significant boost in his workouts. The weights felt lighter, his stamina improved, and most importantly, his muscles began to grow again. Quantitatively, he gained noticeable muscle mass and strength, evidenced by increased bench press and squat numbers. The gains were not just in the numbers; they were visible in the mirror, where a more defined physique began to emerge. Recovery, once a tiresome part of his routine, became more efficient. Muscle soreness diminished, allowing him to train with intensity and frequency previously unattainable. This newfound ability to push his limits without the usual fatigue marked a turning point in Alex's fitness journey.

The long-term impact of peptide use redefined Alex's approach to training. The plateau that once stifled his progress became a steppingstone to new heights. Peptides became an integral part of his training regimen. The motivation that had dwindled returned with vigor, as each session brought him closer to his goals. With the consistent use of peptides, he set new targets, each more ambitious than the last. His confidence soared, not only in his physical capabilities but also in his understanding of how to support his body through science. The integration of peptides into his routine was not a temporary fix but a sustained strategy that aligned with his vision of peak performance. Alex's experience underscores the potential of peptides to revolutionize fitness pursuits, transforming barriers into opportunities for growth and success.

Cognitive Enhancement: Real-Life Nootropic Experiences

Imagine the relentless pace of a typical workday, where the mental fog seems to settle in by mid-morning, and focusing on tasks feels like a Herculean effort. This was the reality for Daniel, a project manager in a high-stakes tech firm. Despite his best efforts, maintaining mental clarity and focus throughout the day was becoming increasingly challenging. The constant need to juggle meetings, deadlines, and complex problem-solving left him feeling mentally exhausted and unproductive. Daniel's drive for excellence pushed him to seek solutions beyond the conventional. His goal was not just to survive the demands but to excel, enhancing his cognitive abilities to match his ambitions and improve overall productivity.

Daniel's exploration led him to the world of nootropic peptides, particularly Noopept and Semax. Noopept, known for its memory-enhancing capabilities, appealed to him as a means to sharpen his recall and cognitive agility. This dipeptide, smaller than many other nootropics, is prized for its ability to cross the blood-brain barrier with ease, acting swiftly to bolster memory functions. Semax, derived from adrenocorticotropic hormone, was selected for its potential to enhance mental clarity and reduce stress-induced cognitive decline. Its mechanism involves modulating neurotransmitter levels, thereby improving concentration and mental resilience. Together, these peptides offered a balanced approach to cognitive enhancement, addressing both memory and focus—two pillars of Daniel's professional performance.

The results were transformative. Daniel reported a marked increase in his ability to concentrate for extended periods. Meetings that once sapped his energy became opportunities to engage and contribute meaningfully. His problem-solving skills saw a noticeable boost, with complex challenges seeming less daunting and more like puzzles to be solved. Objectively, his productivity metrics showed an uptick; tasks were completed more efficiently, and his decision-making process became more streamlined. Colleagues noticed the change, often commenting on his renewed enthusiasm and insight during collaborative sessions. This cognitive renewal did not just foster professional growth but also brought a sense of personal satisfaction and achievement.

The sustainable incorporation of these peptides into Daniel's routine required thoughtful adaptation. Understanding that cognitive health is multifaceted, he balanced the peptide regimen with lifestyle changes. Regular physical exercise became a staple, supporting brain health through increased blood flow and endorphin release. Nutrition played a vital role, with a diet rich in omega-3 fatty acids and antioxidants to nourish the brain. Mindfulness practices, including meditation, complemented the biochemical support provided by the peptides, fostering mental calm and focus. Daniel maintained a journal, tracking cognitive performance and adjusting peptide dosages based on observed effects, ensuring a personalized approach to his cognitive wellness.

Daniel's experience with nootropic peptides illustrates the profound impact they can have on cognitive function when used judiciously and in harmony with other health practices. His story is a testament to the potential of peptides to elevate mental capabilities, offering a path to enhanced productivity and cognitive resilience in the face of modern professional challenges.

Peptides in Stress Management and Recovery

In the bustling city life where the pressure to excel is relentless, stress often becomes an unwelcome companion. Take the case of Karen, a marketing executive whose daily grind began to take a toll on her health. She faced chronic fatigue, a constant sense of being overwhelmed, and persistent sleep disturbances that left her exhausted even after what should have been a full night's rest. The stress-induced health problems were creeping into every corner of her life, affecting her work performance and personal relationships. Sleep, meant to be a refuge, turned into a nightly struggle, with rest elusive and mornings bringing no relief. Karen's quest for a solution led her to explore the potential of peptides to manage stress and enhance recovery, focusing on Thymosin Beta-4 and DSIP (Delta Sleep Inducing Peptide) as her allies.

Thymosin Beta-4, known for its ability to mitigate stress, was a natural choice for Karen's regimen. This peptide helps to modulate the body's stress response, reducing inflammation and promoting healing processes that stress often disrupts. It supports the repair of tissues and organs, offering a foundation for resilience against stress-induced damage. On the other hand, DSIP, a peptide celebrated for its role in promoting restful sleep, was incorporated to address Karen's sleep challenges. DSIP assists in regulating sleep patterns by modulating the neuroendocrine system, promoting a state of relaxation conducive to sleep. Together, these peptides formed a balanced regimen aimed at tackling both the physiological and psychological aspects of stress, providing a comprehensive approach to recovery.

The adoption of this peptide regimen brought about notable changes in Karen's life. She began to experience less stress and more relaxation. Stress markers, often elevated due to chronic stress, showed a decline, signaling a shift towards better stress management. Sleep, once fragmented and insufficient, transformed into a restorative experience. Karen reported longer sleep durations and a deeper quality of rest, waking up refreshed and ready to face the day. The improvement in her sleep quality played a crucial role in enhancing her overall well-being, as sleep is foundational to recovery and stress management. With better rest, Karen found herself more equipped to handle daily challenges with a calm and focused mind.

Integrating peptides into her broader stress management plan was key to sustaining these improvements. Karen combined peptide therapy with mindfulness practices, such as meditation and deep breathing exercises, to reinforce relaxation and mental clarity. These techniques complemented the calming effects of the peptides, creating a synergistic approach to stress relief. Regular monitoring of her stress levels and sleep patterns allowed Karen to adjust her peptide doses as needed, ensuring that her regimen remained effective and aligned with her evolving needs. This adaptability was critical in maintaining the benefits of peptide therapy, as stressors and health needs can fluctuate over time. Through thoughtful integration and continuous evaluation, Karen managed to reclaim her health and balance, illustrating the potential of peptides as a powerful tool in the quest for stress management and recovery.

Personal Insights: Peptides and Emotional Well-being

Amid life's chaos, emotional well-being often feels like a distant goal. This was especially true for Lisa, a 34-year-old graphic designer whose life seemed to be governed by anxiety and unpredictable mood swings. Her emotional health was a rollercoaster, with anxiety peaking at the most inconvenient times, leaving her feeling overwhelmed and unable to focus on her work or enjoy personal interactions. Even simple social gatherings became sources of stress rather than joy. The instability in her mood cast a shadow over her daily life, straining her relationships with colleagues and loved ones. She found herself stuck in a cycle of emotional turmoil, longing for a sense of balance and stability that seemed increasingly out of reach.

In her search for emotional balance, Lisa discovered the potential of peptides, particularly Selank and Oxytocin, to support emotional health. Selank, a synthetic peptide known for its anxiolytic (anxiety-reducing) properties, became a focal point of her approach. It works by modulating neurotransmitter levels, promoting a sense of calm and reducing anxiety without the sedative effects typical of traditional anti-anxiety medications. Meanwhile, Oxytocin, often dubbed the "love hormone," was included for its ability to enhance social bonding and mood. This peptide is naturally released during positive social interactions, contributing to feelings of trust and emotional connection. By incorporating these peptides into her routine, Lisa aimed to address both the anxiety that plagued her and the emotional disconnection she felt from those around her.

The transformation Lisa experienced was profound. Over time, she noticed a marked consistency in her mood, with the peaks and valleys of anxiety smoothing into gentle waves. Her anxiety levels dropped, replaced by a newfound calm that allowed her to engage with the world more fully. Social interactions, once a source of dread, became opportunities for connection and joy. The steadying of her emotional state had a ripple effect, leading to enhanced interpersonal relationships and a richer social life. Friends and family noticed the change, often commenting on her newfound ease and openness. Lisa's work life also benefited; she found herself more focused and productive, able to channel her creativity without the interruptions of anxiety and mood swings.

For Lisa, the journey toward emotional well-being did not stop with peptide therapy. She recognized the importance of integrating these biochemical tools with other emotional health practices. Counseling became a cornerstone of her strategy, providing a space to explore underlying issues and develop coping mechanisms. This therapeutic support complemented the effects of the peptides, offering a holistic approach to emotional health. Mindfulness practices, such as meditation and yoga, were also incorporated, fostering a deeper sense of presence and calm. These practices, alongside regular exercise and a balanced diet, created a foundation for sustained emotional well-being.

The personal growth Lisa experienced through this integrated approach was significant. She became more resilient and better equipped to handle life's challenges with grace and composure. The combination of peptides and holistic practices offered her a path to lasting emotional stability, transforming her daily life from one of struggle to one of balance and fulfillment. Lisa's story highlights the potential of peptides to support emotional health, offering a beacon of hope for those seeking to reclaim their emotional well-being.

Everyday Biohacking: Integrating Peptides into Your Routine

In the ever-evolving world of biohacking, enthusiasts are constantly on the lookout for methods that promise to enhance health and performance. This quest for optimization often leads to the innovative use of peptides, which are embraced by those eager to explore cutting-edge techniques. The motivations behind this choice are varied but centered around the desire to feel and function at their best. Whether it's increasing energy levels, improving mental clarity, or supporting muscle recovery, the appeal lies in the potential to fine-tune one's biology. For many, biohacking is more than a hobby; it's a lifestyle that integrates science with personal health goals, allowing individuals to take proactive control over their well-being.

Incorporating peptides into a daily routine can seem daunting at first, but enthusiasts have found ways to seamlessly weave them into their lives. Morning and evening protocols are popular, with each time of day offering unique benefits. For example, morning use might focus on peptides that boost energy and mental focus, setting a productive tone for the day. Evening protocols, on the other hand, often include peptides that support relaxation and recovery, preparing the body for restful sleep. This thoughtful scheduling ensures that peptides complement the body's natural rhythms, enhancing their effectiveness. By aligning peptide use with daily activities, enthusiasts can experience the benefits without disruption, integrating these compounds as naturally as they might a morning cup of coffee or evening meditation.

The practical benefits of this integration are both tangible and profound. Users often report enhanced energy levels throughout the day, allowing them to approach tasks with renewed vigor and enthusiasm. This boost in energy translates to improved productivity, whether in professional settings or personal pursuits. Focus sharpens, and distractions become easier to manage, leading to more efficient work or study sessions. Beyond productivity, many experience general improvements in their overall sense of well-being, feeling more balanced and in tune with their bodies. The cumulative effect of these benefits is a heightened sense of control over one's health, empowering individuals to pursue their goals with confidence and clarity.

To sustain these benefits, maintaining a consistent and effective peptide routine is crucial. Success hinges on thoughtful planning and adherence to the regimen. Scheduling is key; setting specific times for peptide administration helps create a habit that becomes second nature. For those new to this practice, starting with a simple schedule and gradually adding complexity as comfort and understanding grow can be helpful. Regular evaluation and adjustment are equally important. As the body adapts, needs may change, and protocols should be flexible enough to accommodate these shifts. Keeping a log of peptide use and its effects can provide valuable insights, allowing for informed adjustments that optimize outcomes. This practice fosters a deeper connection with one's health, turning biohacking from a series of experiments into a personalized wellness strategy.

Incorporating peptides into everyday life offers a unique opportunity to explore the frontier of health optimization. By embracing these compounds, individuals can unlock new levels of performance and well-being, enhancing their quality of life in meaningful ways. The stories and strategies shared in this chapter highlight the diverse applications of peptides, showcasing their potential to transform daily routines into powerful tools for personal growth and health enhancement. As we move forward, we'll continue to explore the broader implications of peptide use, delving into advanced biohacking techniques and their impact on long-term wellness.

Chapter 6:
Navigating the Peptide Marketplace

Imagine stepping into a bustling marketplace, vibrant with the hum of possibilities, each stall offering promises of health and vitality. As alluring as this scene might be, it underscores a crucial truth: not all offerings are created equal. When it comes to peptides, the stakes are higher. These powerful molecules hold the key to unlocking potential health benefits, making the quality of your purchase pivotal. Choosing the right source is akin to selecting a trusted jeweler for a precious gem. The right decision can lead to a treasure trove of benefits, while a misstep might invite risks, compromising both safety and efficacy.

Quality can't be overstated when sourcing peptides. Low-quality peptides pose contamination risks, much like a tainted ingredient spoiling an entire recipe. Contaminated peptides can introduce impurities that not only hinder efficacy but also pose serious health threats. Imagine investing time and energy into a regimen, only to discover that the benefits are eroded by impurities. Purity ensures that peptides perform their intended functions effectively, offering the therapeutic benefits they promise. It is imperative to ensure that what you receive is as promised, a pure and potent product ready to engage with your body systems harmoniously.

To navigate this complex landscape, thorough research into potential vendors becomes indispensable. Start by scrutinizing vendor credentials and their industry reputation. A supplier with a solid track record is often synonymous with reliability, akin to a seasoned craftsman known for precision. Look for those who have established their standing over time, as they are likely to uphold stringent quality standards. Customer reviews and testimonials can also serve as invaluable guides. Just as you might consult friends for restaurant recommendations, feedback from other customers provides insight into the vendor's consistency and service quality. It's a way to glean the collective wisdom of past buyers, guiding you toward informed decisions.

Equally important is verifying third-party testing and certifications. Independent verification acts as a seal of approval, much like a certified letter guaranteeing authenticity. Recognized testing laboratories that vouch for a supplier's products lend credibility and assurance. Certificates of Analysis (CoA) are more than just documents; they are proof of purity and potency, transparently outlining the product's composition. A trustworthy supplier will willingly provide these certificates, demonstrating their commitment to transparency and quality. This transparency is a cornerstone of trust, reassuring you that what you are purchasing meets the highest standards.

In assessing a supplier's dedication to quality control, look for compliance with Good Manufacturing Practices (GMP). This adherence is indicative of a commitment to maintaining high standards, akin to a chef ensuring every dish meets the same quality. Regular audits and quality assurance processes further signal a supplier's focus on maintaining product integrity. These practices are the backbone of a reliable supply chain, ensuring that each batch of peptides is consistent in quality and efficacy. A supplier's dedication to these processes reflects their respect for the consumer and the science behind peptides, underscoring their role as facilitators of health and wellness.

Resource List: Trusted Peptide Suppliers

- **Peptide Source Inc.:** Known for stringent quality controls and extensive product testing.
- **Bio-Active Peptides Co.:** Offers a wide range of peptides with detailed CoAs available on request.
- **Pure Peptides Lab:** Specializes in high-purity peptides, adhering to GMP standards.
- **Peptide Solutions:** Provides comprehensive customer support and consultation services.

As you embark on this journey, remember that your choices in the peptide marketplace will directly influence the outcomes you seek. The diligence invested in sourcing quality peptides is not just an exercise in caution; it is a commitment to your health and wellness journey, ensuring that each peptide you introduce into your regimen is a step toward greater vitality and balance.

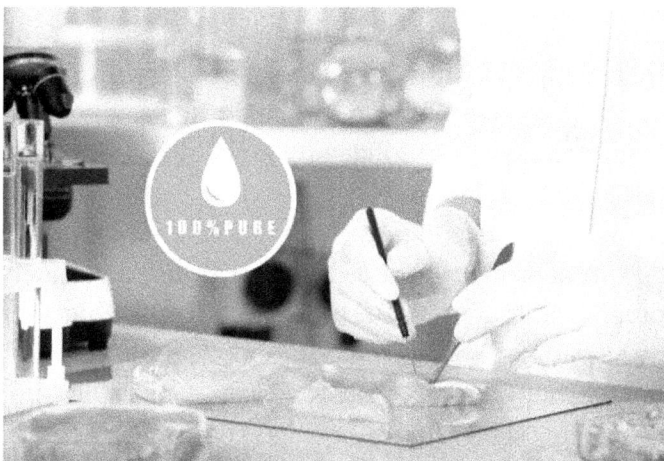

Red Flags and Pitfalls: Avoiding Counterfeit Products

Navigating the intricate landscape of the peptide market requires a keen eye and a healthy dose of skepticism. Counterfeit products, unfortunately, are not uncommon and pose serious risks to both health and wallet. Imagine ordering what you believe to be a pristine product, only to receive something subpar, wrapped in shoddy packaging with labels peeling away. The quality of packaging can be a significant indicator of product authenticity. Genuine products often come with professionally done packaging, clear labeling, and all necessary information prominently displayed. In contrast, counterfeit items might have misspellings, vague product details, or even missing labels altogether. It's akin to buying a luxury handbag only to find the logo askew and the zipper stuck.

Another telltale sign of counterfeit peptides is pricing that seems too good to be true. While everyone loves a bargain, exceptionally low prices should set off alarm bells. Genuine peptides require meticulous manufacturing processes that come at a cost. If a deal seems suspiciously cheap, it might be due to compromised quality or worse, the product could be fake. Think of it like finding a "diamond" ring at a flea market for pennies—it's unlikely to be the real deal.

Beyond pricing and packaging, the lack of batch numbers and traceable information can be a significant red flag. Legitimate products will have batch numbers that allow you to verify the product's origin and manufacturing details. This traceability is crucial for accountability and ensures the product can be traced back through the supply chain. Counterfeit products, on the other hand, often lack these identifiers, making it impossible to confirm their authenticity. The absence of professional contact information is another red flag. Reputable vendors provide clear contact details, allowing you to reach out with questions or concerns. If this information is missing, proceed with caution.

Distinguishing between legitimate and fake products involves more than just examining the surface. Consistency in product appearance and quality is key. Authentic peptides tend to have a uniform appearance, with no discolorations or inconsistencies. Counterfeit products might display variations that suggest poor manufacturing standards. Customer support responsiveness is another crucial factor. Genuine suppliers will have knowledgeable staff ready to assist with inquiries, demonstrating their commitment to customer satisfaction. If you're met with vague responses or a lack of expertise, it could indicate a lack of credibility.

Using counterfeit peptides isn't just a matter of wasting money—it's a health risk. Unverified substances can contain harmful contaminants that pose serious health threats. Without proper regulation and quality control, these products might introduce impurities that can lead to adverse reactions. Beyond health risks, there's the legal aspect to consider. Possessing counterfeit peptides can lead to legal repercussions, as these products might not comply with regulatory standards. It's similar to buying counterfeit currency; while it might seem like a good deal, the consequences are severe.

In this complex market, awareness is your greatest ally. By staying informed and vigilant, you can confidently navigate the peptide landscape. Always prioritize safety and quality, ensuring that the products you choose contribute positively to your health and well-being.

HEALING WITH PEPTIDES: THE ULTIMATE GUIDE TO BIOHACKING YOUR BODY

HELP US GROW WITH YOUR REVIEW!

WE'D LOVE YOUR FEEDBACK!

THANK YOU FOR CHOOSING HEALING WITH PEPTIDES: THE ULTIMATE GUIDE TO BIOHACKING YOUR BODY AS PART OF YOUR HEALTH AND WELLNESS JOURNEY. YOUR FEEDBACK IS INCREDIBLY VALUABLE TO US! IF YOU FOUND THE INSIGHTS AND INFORMATION IN THIS BOOK HELPFUL, WE WOULD GREATLY APPRECIATE IT IF YOU COULD LEAVE A POSITIVE REVIEW. SIMPLY SCAN THE QR CODE BELOW TO SHARE YOUR THOUGHTS. YOUR REVIEW NOT ONLY SUPPORTS US IN REACHING MORE PEOPLE BUT ALSO HELPS TO SPREAD THE MESSAGE OF CUTTING-EDGE WELLNESS AND PEPTIDE-BASED HEALING.

THANK YOU FOR YOUR SUPPORT!

Legal Aspects of Peptide Use: Staying Compliant

Navigating the legal landscape of peptide use requires an understanding of the complex regulatory environment that governs their sale and use. Each country or region may have its own set of rules that classify peptides differently, often as research chemicals rather than supplements. This classification can significantly affect how you purchase and use peptides, as research chemicals are typically intended for laboratory use and not for human consumption. Understanding these distinctions is crucial, as it informs the legal obligations you must adhere to when acquiring peptides. In some jurisdictions, regulations might be more stringent, requiring documentation and proof of intended use. This regulatory framework aims to ensure consumer safety and prevent misuse, making it vital for you to familiarize yourself with the specific laws applicable in your region.

Ensuring compliance with local laws is not just about adhering to regulations but also about protecting yourself from legal repercussions. Consulting local regulatory guidelines can provide clarity and guidance on what is permissible. This might involve reviewing government publications or seeking advice from professionals familiar with the legalities of peptide use. Additionally, keeping thorough documentation of your purchases and usage can serve as evidence of your compliance efforts. This documentation should include invoices, receipts, and any correspondence with suppliers, creating a paper trail that verifies the legitimacy of your transactions. Such records can be invaluable if questions about your peptide use arise, providing transparency and accountability.

In an ever-evolving field like peptides, staying informed about legal changes is paramount. Regulations can shift as new research emerges and as authorities adapt to advancements in peptide science. Monitoring reputable news sources and engaging with professional forums can keep you updated on these changes. These platforms often provide insights from experts and peers, offering a community-based approach to staying informed. Regularly checking these sources ensures that you remain compliant with current laws and are aware of any upcoming changes that could affect your peptide use. Being proactive in this regard can prevent potential legal issues and help you make informed decisions about incorporating peptides into your health regimen.

The consequences of non-compliance with peptide regulations can be severe. Unauthorized use or possession of peptides might result in fines or legal action, tarnishing personal and professional reputations. Legal ramifications can extend beyond financial penalties, potentially affecting your career or professional standing if you are found in violation of regulatory standards. For instance, professionals in healthcare or scientific fields may face disciplinary actions or loss of licensure if caught using peptides illegally. Understanding these risks underscores the importance of adhering to legal guidelines and maintaining transparency in your peptide-related activities. Remaining vigilant and informed about the legal aspects of peptide use is crucial for safeguarding your interests and ensuring that you can continue to benefit from these powerful molecules without legal complications.

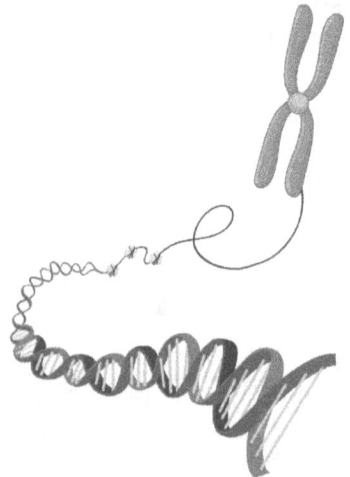

Choosing the Right Supplier: What to Look For

In the world of peptides, finding a reliable supplier can feel like searching for a needle in a haystack. The market is vast, and not every vendor is created equal. When evaluating potential suppliers, certain traits serve as indicators of reliability and trustworthiness. A strong industry presence and history are crucial. Companies with a long-standing reputation often have a proven track record of delivering quality products consistently. They've weathered the ebbs and flows of the market, demonstrating resilience and commitment to their craft. Transparency in business practices and policies is another key trait. Reliable suppliers are upfront about their sourcing, manufacturing processes, and pricing. They provide clear terms of service, leaving little room for ambiguity. This openness builds trust and reassures customers that they are dealing with a reputable company.

Customer service is the backbone of any successful business, and peptide suppliers are no exception. Accessible and knowledgeable customer service can make all the difference in your purchasing experience. Look for suppliers who offer expert advice and consultation, guiding you through product selection and usage. These services signal that the company values customer satisfaction and is invested in your success. Responsive communication channels are equally important. Whether it's through email, phone, or chat, being able to reach a representative easily and receive timely responses is crucial. It ensures that any issues or questions can be addressed swiftly, preventing disruptions in your peptide regimen. This level of support demonstrates a supplier's dedication to maintaining a positive customer relationship.

The range and specialization of products offered by a supplier can also be a deciding factor. A diverse product range indicates that the supplier can cater to various needs, providing options for different health goals and protocols. Whether you're looking for peptides to enhance muscle growth, support cognitive function, or aid in weight management, a supplier with a wide selection is more likely to meet your specific requirements. Specialization in high-demand or niche peptides can also be a plus. Suppliers who focus on specific areas often have a deeper understanding of those products, ensuring higher quality and efficacy. This specialization can provide you with confidence that the peptides you receive are tailored to your particular needs and come with the expertise to back them up.

Supplier policies and guarantees offer an additional layer of assurance when purchasing peptides. A supplier's return and refund policies can speak volumes about their confidence in their products. Fair and transparent policies indicate a willingness to stand behind their offerings, providing peace of mind to customers. If a product doesn't meet your expectations or if there is an issue with your order, knowing that you have the option to return or exchange it is reassuring. These assurances can include guarantees of product purity, potency, and efficacy, backed by robust quality control measures. Such policies highlight the supplier's dedication to maintaining the highest standards and delivering on their promises.

When selecting a peptide supplier, these considerations can guide you toward making an informed and confident choice. A supplier who embodies these qualities is more likely to offer a positive purchasing experience, ensuring that you receive high-quality peptides tailored to your needs. By prioritizing these traits, you can navigate the peptide marketplace with greater clarity and assurance, knowing that you're partnering with a supplier who values quality, transparency, and customer satisfaction. This approach not only enhances your peptide regimen but also contributes to your overall health and wellness journey, empowering you to achieve your goals with confidence and peace of mind.

Storage and Handling: Maintaining Peptide Potency

Imagine you're holding a vial of peptides, a small but potent tool for enhancing your health. The journey of this vial from production to your hand involves meticulous care, and the responsibility now shifts to you to preserve its integrity. Proper storage of peptides is crucial to maintaining their quality and potency. Think of your refrigerator as the guardian of these sensitive molecules. Keeping peptides refrigerated at a consistent temperature of around 4°C (39°F) is recommended for short-term storage, while long-term storage requires even colder conditions, ideally at -20°C (-4°F). Avoid placing them near the refrigerator door, where temperature fluctuations might occur. This ensures they remain stable and effective, much like how a fine wine is best kept in a cellar, away from light and temperature changes.

Light and moisture are the enemies of peptide stability. Store peptides in a dry, dark place to protect them from these degrading elements. Peptides are sensitive to environmental conditions, and exposure can lead to degradation. Use opaque containers or place them in a dark area to shield them from light. Moisture, too, can affect peptide integrity, so ensure that vials are tightly sealed and stored in environments with low humidity. It's akin to safeguarding a precious photograph from fading, keeping it tucked away in an album rather than exposed to the elements.

Handling peptides requires precision and care. When reconstituting peptides, use sterile techniques to avoid contamination. Think of this process as a delicate laboratory procedure, where cleanliness is paramount. Utilize sterile syringes and vials, ensuring all equipment is free from contaminants. Wearing gloves and working in a clean environment can prevent accidental introduction of impurities. The process of reconstitution should be done with steady hands and a clear mind, much like a chef precisely measuring ingredients for a recipe. This careful approach ensures that the peptides remain pure and effective, ready to deliver their intended benefits.

As you inspect your peptides, be on the lookout for signs of degradation. Changes in color or consistency can indicate that a peptide has lost its potency. Clear peptides should remain clear; any cloudiness or the presence of particulates is a warning sign. It's comparable to inspecting produce at the market—if it doesn't look right, it probably isn't. Recognizing these signs early can prevent ineffective or harmful use, ensuring that what you administer is safe and beneficial. This vigilance helps maintain the quality of your regimen, optimizing the effects of peptide therapy.

To extend the shelf life of peptides, minimize their exposure to frequent temperature changes. Each time peptides are exposed to room temperature, their stability is challenged. Avoid leaving them out for extended periods and return them to their proper storage environment promptly. Proper labeling and organization are also key to managing your peptide supply efficiently. Label vials with the date of reconstitution and any relevant details, much like a well-organized kitchen pantry. This practice ensures that you can easily access and identify each peptide, reducing the risk of using expired or compromised products. By implementing these strategies, you maximize the potential of peptides, supporting your health goals with precision and effectiveness.

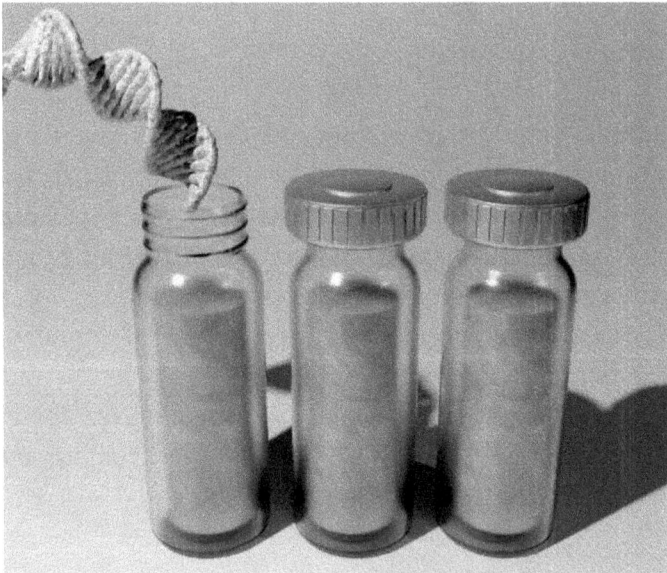

Navigating the peptide marketplace isn't just about choosing the right supplier; it's also about managing your finances to sustain long-term health investments. Creating a financial plan for peptide purchases starts with understanding your specific health goals. Are you aiming to boost muscle growth, enhance cognitive function, or perhaps improve skin health? Prioritizing these goals helps you allocate resources efficiently. Begin by listing the peptides that align with your objectives, then factor in their costs against your monthly or yearly budget. Consider this strategy as akin to meal planning—knowing what you need ahead of time ensures you don't overspend or purchase unnecessary items.

Quality over quantity is a guiding principle here. While it might be tempting to stock up on a variety of peptides, focusing on fewer, high-quality options often yields better results. Think of it like choosing a few key pieces for your wardrobe rather than buying an abundance of fast fashion that won't last. Investing in quality ensures that the peptides you use are effective, reducing the likelihood of needing to buy more in an attempt to achieve desired outcomes. This approach not only saves money in the long run but also enhances the efficacy of your health regimen.

To maximize value without compromising quality, explore cost-saving strategies that can make the use of peptide more affordable. Bulk purchasing is one option, with discounts often available for larger orders. This can significantly lower costs per unit, much like buying staple foods in bulk at a warehouse club. However, ensure you can store peptides properly to maintain their potency. Subscription services offer another avenue for savings, providing regular shipments at reduced rates. These services not only help manage costs but also ensure a steady supply, preventing interruptions in your peptide regimen. It's similar to having a magazine subscription—consistent, reliable, and often less expensive than buying individual issues.

Balancing cost with quality assurance means avoiding the false economy of cheap, low-quality products. While these might seem like a bargain, they often lack the purity and potency needed for effective results. Investing in reputable suppliers ensures that you're getting value for your money, much like buying from a trusted brand known for durability. There is truth in the old adage, "you get what you pay for." Long-term, this strategy saves you from the potential pitfalls of ineffective or harmful products. It's important to evaluate the cost-effectiveness of your peptide protocols regularly. Are you achieving the desired results, or is there room for improvement? Adjustments might be needed as your health goals evolve or as new research emerges, guiding you to refine your peptide choices.

Planning for long-term peptide use involves a commitment to sustainability in your health practices. Regularly reviewing and adjusting your peptide budget ensures that it aligns with both your current needs and future goals. This proactive approach helps you adapt to changes, whether in your financial situation or health objectives, and creates a flexible framework that accommodates growth and change. It's like maintaining a garden; regular care and adjustments keep it thriving, allowing you to reap the benefits season after season.

In conclusion, navigating the peptide marketplace is more than just making purchases; it's about creating a sustainable, effective strategy that supports your health goals. By balancing quality with affordability, leveraging cost-saving strategies, and regularly evaluating your approach, you can ensure that peptide use remains a beneficial part of your wellness routine. As we move forward, the next chapter will delve into advanced biohacking techniques, exploring how peptides can be integrated with other health optimization strategies for even greater results.

Chapter 7:
Advanced Biohacking Techniques

Picture yourself in a bustling city park on a crisp morning, armed with a smartwatch and headphones. You're not just tracking your steps or listening to music; you're actively engaging in a sophisticated biohacking routine. This includes monitoring heart rate, tracking sleep patterns, and, importantly, optimizing your health with peptides. In recent years, biohacking has evolved from simple lifestyle tweaks to a complex interplay of science and technology, allowing us to take control of our health like never before. Peptides, those small but mighty chains of amino acids, have become a crucial component in this modern health revolution. By integrating peptides with traditional biohacking practices, you can enhance your body's normal capabilities, improve recovery times, and even boost cognitive function.

Integrating peptides with other biohacking methods can significantly amplify your health efforts. For instance, pairing peptides with intermittent fasting can yield remarkable results. Intermittent fasting, the practice of cycling between periods of fasting and eating, can enhance the efficacy of peptides by improving metabolic flexibility. Peptides like Ipamorelin, which boosts growth hormone levels, can further augment fasting benefits by promoting fat loss and muscle preservation. This synergistic effect not only optimizes body composition but also supports cellular repair processes during fasting windows. Cold exposure triggers the release of norepinephrine, a hormone that works in tandem with peptides to reduce pain and inflammation. By leveraging these combined effects, you can accelerate recovery and enhance resilience, paving the way for improved performance and well-being.

The integration of peptides with technology presents new opportunities for health optimization. Wearable devices, like fitness trackers and smartwatches, can monitor the effects of peptides in real time, providing valuable insights into your body's responses. These devices track metrics such as heart rate variability, sleep quality, and activity levels, offering a comprehensive view of your health. When combined with peptide therapy, these insights allow for precise adjustments to your routine, ensuring that you maximize the benefits of your interventions. Biofeedback systems take this a step further, enabling real-time adjustments based on physiological data. By receiving immediate feedback on how your body responds to peptides and other biohacking strategies, you can refine your approach to achieve optimal outcomes. This integration of technology and peptides empowers you to take a proactive role in managing your health, aligning your interventions with your body's unique needs.

Achieving the best results from biohacking requires a holistic approach that balances physical, mental, and emotional health. Peptides can play a crucial role in this comprehensive strategy by supporting various aspects of well-being. For instance, peptides known for their cognitive-enhancing properties can improve focus and mental clarity, allowing you to perform at your best in daily tasks. Meanwhile, peptides that support immune function can enhance your body's resilience, reducing the likelihood of illness and promoting overall vitality. By combining peptides with practices that support mental health, such as mindfulness or meditation, you foster a balanced approach to wellness that addresses all aspects of your health. This holistic perspective is essential for sustaining long-term well-being and achieving your health goals.

To seamlessly incorporate peptides into your biohacking routine, consider creating a schedule that aligns with your daily activities. Begin by identifying specific health goals and selecting the peptides that support those objectives. For example, if your goal is to improve athletic performance, focus on peptides that enhance recovery and muscle growth. Integrate these peptides into your routine by scheduling administration around your workouts or recovery periods. Additionally, explore protocols that combine peptides with other biohacking methods for synergistic effects. For instance, you might pair peptides with morning cold exposure sessions or use them as part of your pre-sleep routine to enhance recovery overnight. By thoughtfully integrating peptides into your lifestyle, you create a comprehensive biohacking strategy that maximizes your health potential.

Interactive Element: Biohacking Protocol Checklist

- Identify Goals: Determine your primary health objectives (e.g., fat loss, cognitive enhancement, recovery).
- Select Peptides: Choose peptides that align with your goals based on their specific benefits.
- Create a Schedule: Plan peptide administration around daily activities for consistency and effectiveness.
- Combine Methods: Integrate peptides with other biohacking practices, such as fasting or tech tracking.
- Monitor Progress: Use technology to track results and adjust your protocol as needed for optimal outcomes.

As you continue to explore the potential of peptides in your biohacking journey, remember that the key to success lies in personalization and adaptability. Tailor your approach to meet your unique needs and remain open to experimenting with different methods to discover what works best for you. By embracing the evolving landscape of biohacking, you empower yourself to achieve new levels of health and wellness.

Peptides and Nutrigenomics: Personalized Nutrition Plans

Imagine being able to tailor your diet based on your unique genetic makeup. This concept, known as nutrigenomics, is revolutionizing how we approach nutrition and health. By understanding how your genes influence nutritional needs, you can create a personalized diet that aligns with your body's specific requirements. Peptides play a vital role in this personalized approach by acting as modulators in the intricate dance of metabolism. Genetic variations can significantly impact how your body processes nutrients, affecting everything from metabolic rate to nutrient absorption. For example, certain genetic markers might make you more efficient at metabolizing carbohydrates, while others could predispose you to better fat utilization. These insights allow for a nutritional strategy that is as unique as your DNA, providing the blueprint for optimal health.

Peptides can guide these dietary interventions by enhancing nutrient absorption and optimizing metabolic processes. For instance, peptides like BPC-157 and TB-500 not only promote healing and reduce inflammation but also improve nutrient uptake, ensuring that your body gets the most out of the food you consume. Imagine your digestive system as a bustling marketplace, with peptides acting as skilled negotiators who ensure that nutrients are absorbed efficiently and distributed where they're needed most. Additionally, peptides can help customize macronutrient ratios based on feedback from your body's responses. If you're genetically predisposed to better utilize fats, incorporating peptides that enhance fat metabolism can amplify these benefits, leading to improved energy levels and weight management.

Genetic testing can further refine peptide use, providing precision that transforms your health strategy from a one-size-fits-all to a tailor-made approach. By examining specific genes that influence peptide efficacy, you can identify which peptides will work best for you. For example, certain genetic markers might indicate a predisposition for better response to peptides that enhance muscle growth, guiding your choice of supplementation. Understanding these interactions allows you to align peptide protocols with your genetic profile, optimizing their benefits. Imagine a world where your genetic code acts as a guidebook, revealing the most effective pathways to achieve your health goals. This integration of genetic insights and peptide therapy creates a potent synergy that enhances your body's natural capabilities.

Consider a hypothetical scenario illustrating the power of personalized nutrition with peptides. Meet Laura, a 35-year-old professional who struggles with energy fluctuations and weight management. After undergoing genetic testing, she discovers that her body is more efficient at metabolizing fats rather than carbohydrates. Armed with this knowledge, Laura adjusts her macronutrient intake, focusing on healthy fats while incorporating peptides like CJC-1295 to boost growth hormone production and enhance fat metabolism. Her meal plan includes avocado, nuts, and olive oil, paired with peptide supplementation to optimize her energy levels and support her fitness goals. Over time, Laura experiences sustained energy throughout the day, improved focus, and a gradual shift in body composition, showcasing the transformative potential of personalized nutrition.

Case Study: Personalized Peptide Nutrition Plan

- **Client Profile:** John is a 50-year-old man with a family history of type 2 diabetes.
- **Genetic Insights:** Genetic testing reveals a predisposition for insulin resistance.
- **Peptide Intervention:** John incorporates Ipamorelin and GHRP-6 to enhance insulin sensitivity and support metabolic health.
- **Dietary Adjustments:** Emphasizes a diet rich in fiber, lean proteins, and healthy fats, reducing refined carbohydrates.
- **Outcome:** Improved blood sugar levels, increased energy, and weight loss over six months.

This personalized plan illustrates the profound impact of aligning peptides and nutrition with genetic insights, offering a glimpse into the future of health optimization. By embracing the science of nutrigenomics and the targeted action of peptides, you unlock new dimensions of health potential.

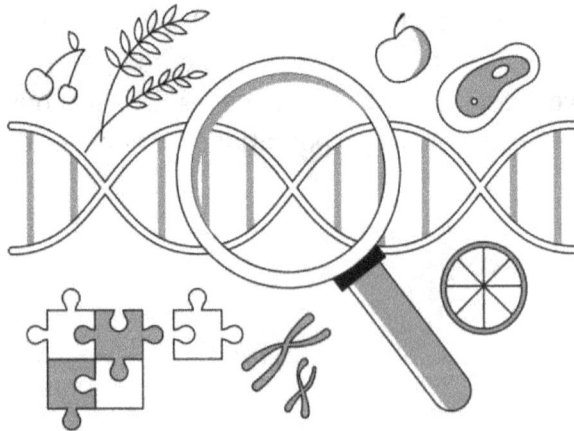

NUTRIGENOMICS

Peptides and Hormone Optimization: Balancing Your Endocrine System

Imagine your endocrine system as a finely tuned orchestra, where each hormone plays a crucial role in maintaining harmony within your body. Peptides are the skilled conductors ensuring that each section performs flawlessly, guiding the flow of hormones to achieve optimal balance. One of the most significant areas where peptides exert their influence is in the regulation of thyroid function. The thyroid gland, a butterfly-shaped gland located in your neck, is responsible for producing hormones that regulate metabolism, energy levels, and overall vitality. Peptides can enhance thyroid function by modulating the release of thyroid-stimulating hormone (TSH), ensuring that your metabolism operates efficiently and your energy levels remain stable. By supporting thyroid health, peptides offer a pathway to improved well-being and vitality, helping to maintain the body's natural rhythm.

In addition to thyroid regulation, peptides play a crucial role in managing cortisol levels, the hormone often referred to as the "stress hormone." Cortisol is released in response to stress, preparing your body to face challenges. However, chronic stress can lead to elevated cortisol levels, which can disrupt sleep, lower immunity, and contribute to weight gain. Peptides, such as Thymosin Beta-4, can help regulate cortisol production, promoting a more balanced stress response. This regulation not only supports mental and emotional well-being but also enhances physical health by reducing inflammation and promoting tissue repair. By keeping cortisol in check, peptides help mitigate the negative effects of stress, fostering resilience and stability in the face of life's challenges.

Peptides interact with various hormonal pathways to modulate hormone levels with precision. One notable example is their effect on insulin sensitivity. Insulin, a hormone produced by the pancreas, regulates blood sugar levels. Peptides like GLP-1 analogs can enhance insulin sensitivity, making cells more responsive to insulin. This improvement can help prevent insulin resistance, a precursor to type 2 diabetes, by ensuring that glucose is efficiently utilized for energy rather than stored as fat. Peptides also influence the balance of testosterone and estrogen, two hormones vital for reproductive health and overall well-being. By modulating these hormone levels, peptides can support muscle growth, enhance libido, and maintain bone density, contributing to a healthier, more vibrant life.

The benefits of using peptides for endocrine health are numerous and far-reaching. By promoting hormonal harmony, peptides can improve energy levels, stabilize mood, and enhance reproductive health. Imagine waking up each day feeling energized and focused, with a sense of balance that permeates every aspect of your life as you are ready to grasp the day. Peptides make this a reality by supporting the body's natural hormone production and regulation. For individuals experiencing hormonal imbalances, peptides offer a targeted approach to restoring equilibrium and improving quality of life. The enhancement of reproductive health is particularly noteworthy, as balanced hormones are essential for fertility, sexual function, and overall vitality. By optimizing hormone levels, peptides provide a means of achieving hormonal harmony and fostering a healthy, fulfilling life.

Implementing hormone-focused protocols with peptides requires careful consideration and monitoring. Begin by identifying specific hormonal imbalances and selecting peptides that target these issues. For instance, if you're experiencing low energy and mood swings due to thyroid dysfunction, consider incorporating peptides that support thyroid health, such as those that modulate TSH levels. Similarly, for stress-related hormonal imbalances, focus on peptides that regulate cortisol production. Monitoring hormonal changes with peptide use is essential to ensure efficacy and safety. Regular blood tests and consultations with healthcare professionals can help track progress and make necessary adjustments to your peptide regimen. By tailoring peptide protocols to your unique hormonal needs, you can achieve a balanced endocrine system that supports your overall health and well-being.

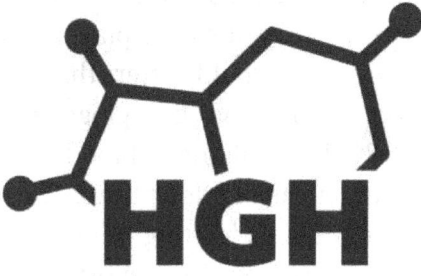

HGH

Enhancing Athletic Performance with Peptides: Legal Strategies

Imagine standing at the starting line of a race, the anticipation palpable, sweat trickling down your brow. The world of sports is fiercely competitive, with athletes continuously seeking that extra edge to outperform their peers. In this quest for excellence, peptides have emerged as a powerful tool for enhancing athletic performance. But with great power comes the need for responsible use. The World Anti-Doping Agency (WADA) plays a pivotal role in ensuring a level playing field, setting clear regulations for peptide use among athletes. WADA's guidelines are designed to prevent unfair advantages while safeguarding the health and integrity of sports. As an athlete or sports enthusiast, it's crucial to familiarize yourself with these regulations to ensure compliance and avoid potential repercussions.

Among the peptides that have garnered attention for their performance-enhancing properties is BPC-157. Known for its ability to accelerate injury recovery, BPC-157 aids in the healing of muscles, tendons, and ligaments. Imagine a soccer player recovering from a torn ligament who can return to the field faster, thanks to the regenerative powers of this peptide. By promoting angiogenesis—the formation of new blood vessels—BPC-157 enhances blood flow to injured areas, speeding up recovery and reducing downtime. This accelerated healing process is invaluable for athletes looking to maintain their competitive edge and minimize time away from their sport. However, it's important to note that while some peptides are permitted for recovery, others are banned by WADA for their performance-enhancing effects. Understanding which peptides are allowed and which are prohibited is essential for athletes to remain compliant with regulations.

Peptides not only aid in recovery but also significantly enhance training outcomes. They promote muscle growth and improve endurance, allowing athletes to push their limits and achieve new personal bests. Consider peptides that stimulate the release of growth hormone, such as GHRP-6, which can increase muscle mass and reduce body fat. For an athlete striving to enhance strength and power, these peptides can be a game-changer. They work by increasing the body's natural production of growth hormone, leading to improved muscle synthesis and faster recovery times. This means that athletes can train harder, recover quicker, and perform better in their chosen sport. However, the use of such peptides must be carefully managed to ensure alignment with ethical and legal standards.

Maintaining integrity and legality in peptide use is paramount for athletes. Collaboration with sports professionals, such as coaches and medical experts, ensures that peptide protocols are tailored to individual needs while adhering to regulatory guidelines. This collaboration provides athletes with the support and expertise needed to use peptides safely and effectively. Transparency in supplementation is also crucial. Keeping detailed records of peptide usage, including dosages and administration schedules, not only promotes accountability but also aids in the event of any regulatory inquiries. Athletes should also stay informed about any updates to WADA's list of prohibited substances, as regulations can change over time.

In the world of competitive sports, where every millisecond counts, peptides offer a promising avenue for enhancing performance and recovery. Yet, the responsibility lies with athletes to use these tools ethically and within the confines of the law. By understanding WADA regulations, choosing legal peptides, and working with trusted professionals, athletes can leverage the benefits of peptides to elevate their performance while upholding the integrity of their sport. The path to excellence is paved with dedication, discipline, and the judicious use of science, ensuring that athletic achievements are celebrated for their authenticity and hard work.

Peptides and Adaptogens: A Combined Approach to Stress

Imagine you're navigating a demanding work week, juggling deadlines, and personal commitments. Your body's stress response is on high alert, ready to tackle challenges but also susceptible to burnout. Here, a combined approach using peptides and adaptogens can be transformative. Adaptogens, like Ashwagandha, have long been valued in traditional medicine for their ability to enhance the body's resilience to stress. They work by modulating the stress response, helping you remain calm and focused. Peptides, on the other hand, play a crucial role in supporting physiological functions that are often compromised under stress, such as adrenal functions. The adrenal glands are responsible for producing stress hormones like cortisol. When stress becomes chronic, these glands can become overworked, leading to fatigue and hormonal imbalances. Peptides can support adrenal health by optimizing hormone production and release, ensuring that your body maintains balance even under pressure.

The synergy between peptides and adaptogens lies in their complementary mechanisms. While adaptogens like Ashwagandha work to calm the mind and stabilize mood, peptides enhance the body's internal processes, fostering resilience from within. This dual action can lead to balanced cortisol levels, improved sleep quality, and a more robust immune system. Consider the analogy of a car engine; adaptogens fine-tune the emotional controls, while peptides ensure the engine itself runs smoothly and efficiently. This comprehensive approach allows you to handle stressors effectively without depleting your resources or compromising your health.

Integrating both peptides and adaptogens into your daily routine can elevate your stress management strategy. Start your day with a calming tea infused with adaptogens, setting a peaceful tone. As you progress through the day, incorporate peptides known for their stress-reducing properties, such as those that support adrenal function. Timing and dosage are key to maximizing their benefits. For example, taking adaptogens in the morning can help prepare your body for daily stressors, while peptides might be more effective when taken later in the day to aid recovery and maintain hormonal balance. A sample routine could involve a morning meditation session with Ashwagandha tea, followed by a peptide supplement post-lunch to sustain energy and focus. As evening approaches, a calming ritual with adaptogens can signal to your body that it's time to wind down, promoting restful sleep.

To ensure optimal synergy, consider the specific needs of your body and lifestyle. If you face intense mental challenges, focus on adaptogens known for cognitive support. For physical stress, peptides that support muscle recovery and hormone balance may be more beneficial. The beauty of this combined approach is its adaptability; you can tailor it to fit your unique stressors and health goals. By taking a proactive stance, you create a personalized framework that not only addresses immediate stress but also builds long-term resilience. This strategy not only enhances your ability to manage stress but also enriches your overall well-being, allowing you to thrive in the face of life's demands. The potential of combining peptides and adaptogens is vast, offering a pathway to a more balanced and fulfilling life.

Cutting-Edge Innovations: The Future of Peptide Research

Peptide research is a dynamic field, constantly evolving with discoveries and technologies that push boundaries. One of the most exciting trends in this domain is the development of novel synthetic peptides. These are engineered to mimic or enhance natural peptides, offering precise control over biological processes. Unlike their natural counterparts, synthetic peptides can be tailored to target specific receptors with high affinity, improving their efficacy and reducing potential side effects. This customization allows for the creation of peptides that are not only more potent but also more stable, overcoming limitations such as rapid degradation in the body. Researchers are exploring these synthetic peptides for a variety of applications, from advanced wound healing to targeted cancer therapies. The ability to design peptides with specific actions opens new avenues for treating complex diseases, offering hope where traditional therapies may have fallen short.

Breakthroughs in peptide technology are further enhancing their delivery and efficacy, making them more accessible and effective for therapeutic use. One such innovation is the use of nanoparticle delivery systems. These tiny carriers protect peptides from degradation, allowing them to reach their target sites intact and with greater precision. Imagine nanoparticles as protective capsules, safeguarding peptides as they navigate the body's complex environment. This technology not only increases the bioavailability of peptides but also enables controlled release, ensuring a sustained therapeutic effect. The precision of nanoparticle delivery minimizes the risk of off-target effects, improving safety and efficacy. Researchers are harnessing this technology to develop peptide-based treatments that are more consistent and reliable, paving the way for new medical applications.

The future of peptide research holds immense promise, particularly in the realms of personalized medicine and gene therapy. Personalized medicine involves tailoring treatments to individual genetic profiles, and peptides are uniquely suited to this approach due to their specificity and adaptability. By integrating genetic insights with peptide therapy, healthcare providers can design treatment plans that are highly customized, improving outcomes and minimizing adverse effects. Peptides are also being explored in gene therapy, where they can be used to deliver genetic material to cells, correcting mutations at their source. This approach has the potential to revolutionize the treatment of genetic disorders, providing long-term solutions rather than temporary relief. As research progresses, we can anticipate the emergence of peptide therapies that are as unique as the individuals they are designed to help.

Staying informed about these advancements is crucial for anyone interested in the potential of peptides. Following key research institutions and publications can provide valuable insights into the latest discoveries and trends. Engaging with the scientific community through conferences and online forums is another way to keep abreast of new developments, fostering a deeper understanding of the field. For those interested in contributing to this exciting area of research or participating in clinical trials or studies can offer firsthand experience with cutting-edge therapies. By staying engaged, you not only enhance your own knowledge but also become part of a movement that is reshaping the landscape of health and medicine. Peptide research is not just about treating diseases; it's about enhancing quality of life and unlocking new possibilities for human health.

Chapter 8:
Expert Insights and Resources

On a sunny afternoon, I found myself in a bustling conference center, surrounded by some of the most brilliant minds in peptide research. The excitement in the air was palpable as experts from around the world gathered to discuss the latest advancements in the field. Among them was Dr. John Smith, a renowned peptide biochemist, who shared his insights on the evolution of peptide science. Dr. Smith spoke passionately about the breakthroughs in peptide delivery systems, highlighting how these innovations could revolutionize therapeutic applications. He explained that advances in nanotechnology are paving the way for more efficient and targeted delivery methods, allowing peptides to reach specific cells with unprecedented precision. This, he said, could potentially open new doors for treating diseases that were previously deemed untouchable.

In a separate session, I had the privilege of speaking with Dr. Emily Chen, a leading expert in the therapeutic applications of peptides. Dr. Chen has dedicated her career to exploring how peptides can be integrated into modern medicine. She explained that peptides are increasingly recognized for their role in personalized medicine, where treatments are tailored to the individual's unique genetic makeup. This approach promises to improve treatment outcomes and reduce side effects, making healthcare more efficient and effective. According to Dr. Chen, one of the most exciting prospects is the development of peptides that can specifically target diseased cells, minimizing harm to healthy tissue and revolutionizing cancer treatment.

As the conference progressed, I gathered practical advice from experienced practitioners who have successfully integrated peptides into clinical settings. They shared best practices for using peptides in therapy, emphasizing the importance of precise dosing and patient monitoring. One practitioner noted the common challenges in peptide application, such as stability and storage, and offered solutions to overcome these hurdles. He recommended using advanced formulation techniques to enhance peptide stability and suggested formal training for healthcare providers to ensure proper administration. These insights underscored the importance of a meticulous approach to peptide therapy, highlighting the need for ongoing education and adaptation.

The role of peptides in modern medicine is undeniably significant. As we continue to unravel their potential, the impact of peptide research on healthcare outcomes becomes increasingly apparent. Peptides offer promising solutions for a variety of therapeutic areas, from metabolic disorders to infectious diseases. They act as hormones, growth factors, and neurotransmitters, providing targeted treatments that are both effective and versatile. In the realm of personalized medicine, peptides play a crucial role in tailoring therapies to individual needs, addressing the unique challenges that each patient presents. This personalized approach not only enhances the efficacy of treatments but also reduces the risk of adverse effects, offering a more holistic and patient-centered model of care.

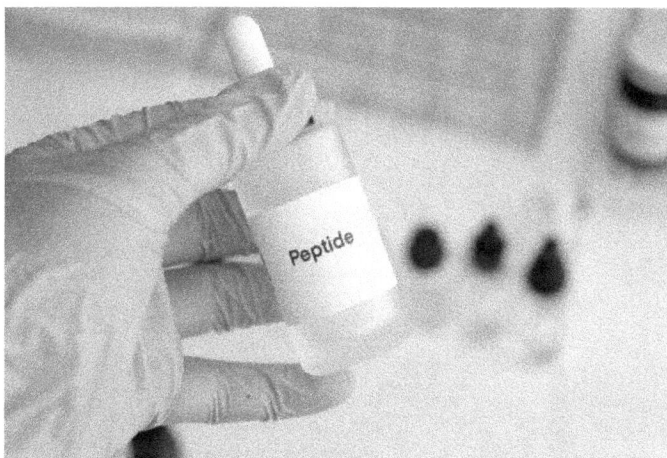

The future of peptides is bright, with anticipated breakthroughs in delivery systems and new therapeutic targets on the horizon. Researchers are exploring novel ways to enhance the bioavailability and stability of peptides, ensuring that they remain effective throughout the treatment process. The development of synthetic peptides that mimic natural ones is also gaining traction, offering more options for therapeutic intervention. As these advancements continue to unfold, the promise of peptides in modern medicine grows, heralding a new era of healthcare innovation that holds the potential to transform patient outcomes and improve quality of life across the globe.

Expert Roundtable: Key Takeaways

- Dr. John Smith: Emphasizes advances in peptide delivery systems and their potential to revolutionize disease treatment.

- Dr. Emily Chen: Highlights peptides' role in personalized medicine, improving treatment precision and reducing side effects.

- Practitioners' Advice: Focus on precise dosing, advanced formulation techniques for stability, and continuous education for effective peptide therapy.

The Latest Research: Staying Updated in the Peptide World

In the ever-evolving landscape of peptide research, recent studies continue to illuminate the potential these compounds hold in medicine and wellness. One of the most exciting developments is the progress made in clinical trials assessing peptide efficacy across various applications. These trials have shown promising results, particularly in chronic disease management, where peptides have demonstrated the ability to modulate disease pathways effectively. For instance, the use of novel peptide analogs has opened new avenues for treating conditions like type 2 diabetes and cardiovascular diseases. These analogs, designed to improve stability and bioavailability, provide a more sustained therapeutic effect, reducing the frequency of administration and enhancing patient compliance. The implications of these findings are profound, suggesting that peptides could soon become a cornerstone in the toolkit for managing chronic illnesses.

Recent discoveries have further highlighted innovations in peptide synthesis techniques, which play a crucial role in advancing therapeutic applications. Advances in synthetic biology and chemical engineering have allowed for the creation of peptides with enhanced properties, such as increased resistance to enzymatic degradation and improved membrane permeability. These improvements address some of the traditional challenges associated with peptide drugs, such as poor in vivo stability, thereby expanding their potential uses in clinical settings. As a result, we can expect to see more peptides being developed for a wider range of therapeutic targets, including those that were previously considered difficult to treat with conventional drugs.

To stay informed about these cutting-edge developments, consider subscribing to reputable journals like "Peptide Science." This journal, along with others in the field, regularly publishes groundbreaking research and reviews that can deepen your understanding of peptide science. Additionally, databases such as PubMed provide access to a vast repository of scientific papers, allowing you to explore the latest findings at your convenience. Engaging with these resources not only keeps you updated but also offers insights into the direction of future research, helping you anticipate emerging trends and innovations.

Active participation in the scientific community can further enhance your understanding and engagement with the world of peptides. Attending conferences and webinars focused on peptide research is an excellent way to connect with experts and peers while gaining firsthand knowledge of the latest advancements. These events often feature presentations from leading researchers and provide a platform for discussing new ideas and technologies. Joining professional organizations, such as the American Peptide Society, can also be beneficial. Membership in such organizations offers access to exclusive resources and networking opportunities, fostering collaboration and exchange of knowledge among members. Engaging with these communities allows you to contribute to the ongoing dialogue in peptide research, keeping you at the forefront of this dynamic field.

Building a Support Network: Communities and Forums

In the digital age, finding like-minded individuals interested in peptides has never been easier. Online communities are vibrant spaces where knowledge is shared, questions are answered, and experiences are exchanged. Platforms like Reddit host several groups focused on peptide discussions, where enthusiasts and novices alike gather to discuss everything from the latest research to personal experiences with peptide protocols. These forums provide a wealth of information, often featuring discussions moderated by knowledgeable enthusiasts who can guide newcomers through the complexities of peptide use. Similarly, Facebook hosts numerous communities dedicated to biohacking, where members post their successes, challenges, and insights into how peptides have impacted their health and wellness journeys. These groups offer more than just information; they provide a sense of belonging, where you can connect with others who share your interest in health optimization.

Engaging with these online communities offers numerous benefits. First, they provide a platform for exchanging practical tips and success stories. Members often share their peptide protocols, offering insights into what has worked for them and what hasn't. This exchange of information can be invaluable, as it allows you to learn from others' experiences and adapt their strategies to suit your own needs. Additionally, these communities offer peer support and accountability. When embarking on a new health regimen, having a network of supportive individuals can make a significant difference. They can provide encouragement, offer advice when challenges arise, and celebrate your successes, making the process feel less isolating and more achievable. By participating in these communities, you gain access to a collective wisdom that can enhance your understanding and application of peptides.

However, navigating these communities requires discernment to ensure you're receiving credible information. It's important to evaluate the credibility of those sharing advice, as not all information is accurate or safe. Look for community leaders who demonstrate proven expertise, provide sources for their claims, and encourage critical thinking. Be wary of discussions that make vague sweeping claims without evidence, or those that promote unsafe practices. Red flags include forums where members discourage consulting healthcare professionals or promote products without discussing potential risks or side effects. By approaching these communities with a critical eye, you can benefit from the wealth of knowledge they offer while avoiding misinformation.

Active participation is key to getting the most out of these communities. Contributing your insights and experiences not only enriches the community but also enhances your own learning. Sharing your personal peptide protocols and the outcomes you've experienced can provide valuable information for others who may be considering similar approaches. Initiating discussions on emerging peptide topics can also stimulate conversation and encourage others to share their knowledge. This collaborative environment fosters a culture of continuous learning and improvement, where members support each other in their pursuit of health and wellness goals.

Community Engagement Checklist

- Join Multiple Forums: **Explore** different platforms to find communities that resonate with your interests and values.
- Evaluate Credibility: **Look** for communities with knowledgeable moderators who provide evidence-based information.
- Engage Actively: **Share** your experiences and insights to contribute to the collective learning of the community.
- Stay Informed: **Regularly** check for updates and participate in discussions to stay engaged and informed.
- Be Open-Minded: **Approach** new ideas with curiosity but maintain a critical perspective to discern credible information.

Connecting with others in these communities provides an opportunity to expand your knowledge, gain support, and contribute to the shared goal of optimizing health through peptides. This interconnectedness fosters a sense of camaraderie, where members learn from each other and grow together in their biohacking endeavors.

Recommended Reading and Resources: Deepening Your Knowledge

Imagine sitting in a cozy corner with a steaming cup of tea, surrounded by a wealth of knowledge waiting to be explored. There's something profoundly enriching about diving into a book that opens new worlds of understanding, especially in a field as dynamic as peptide science. "The Peptide Protocols" by Dr. Jane Doe is a treasure trove of information, offering detailed insights into the practical applications of peptides in health and wellness. This book is a must-read for anyone eager to deepen their understanding of how these powerful molecules can be integrated into daily routines for optimal health benefits. It covers a range of topics, from the basics of peptide biology to advanced therapeutic strategies, making it an invaluable resource for both beginners and seasoned enthusiasts.

For those who prefer a more interactive experience, multimedia resources provide a versatile way to learn. Podcasts featuring leading peptide experts dive into discussions about the latest research, offering listeners the chance to absorb complex information in an accessible format. Videos and online courses go further, providing visual learners with detailed explanations and demonstrations of peptide applications. Many courses offer certifications in peptide science, adding a layer of credibility and depth to your knowledge. These resources cater to various learning styles, ensuring that you can find a format that resonates with you and fits into your lifestyle. Whether you're commuting, exercising, or simply relaxing at home, these multimedia tools offer a convenient way to stay informed and engaged.

Reputable websites and databases are another cornerstone of continued learning. The European Peptide Society, for instance, offers a wealth of resources that are both reliable and up-to-date. Accessing platforms like ResearchGate can connect you with a global community of scientists and researchers, allowing you to explore cutting-edge studies and publications. These platforms provide a space where you can read and discuss the latest findings, staying abreast of the continuous advancements in peptide research. These sites not only keep you informed but also offer opportunities to engage with experts and peers, fostering a collaborative environment for learning and discovery. By regularly visiting these sites, you can ensure that your knowledge remains current and comprehensive.

In a fast-paced world where new information is constantly emerging, ongoing education is not just beneficial—it's crucial. Settingaside dedicated time each week for reading and research can help you stay aligned with the latest advancements. Engage in lifelonglearning practices by attending workshops, webinars, and lectures that broaden your horizons and deepen your expertise. Thiscommitment to education empowers you to make informed decisions about your health and wellness, ensuring that you can adapt tonew developments with confidence. By embracing continuous learning, you cultivate a mindset that is open to innovation and growth,positioning yourself at the forefront of the peptide field. This proactive approach allows you to harness the benefits of peptides fully, enhancing your well-being and enriching your life.

Beyond Peptides: Exploring Complementary Therapies

In the realm of health optimization, the integration of complementary therapies with peptide use can create a powerful synergy that enhances overall well-being. Acupuncture, a time-honored practice, is one such therapy that can amplify the benefits of peptides. By stimulating specific points of the body, acupuncture can improve circulation and boost the body's natural healing processes, creating an environment where peptides can work more efficiently. This ancient method, when used alongside peptides, can help alleviate chronic pain and reduce inflammation, offering a holistic approach to managing health issues. Imagine combining the targeted healing capabilities of peptides with the wide-reaching benefits of acupuncture—it's like supercharging your body's ability to repair and rejuvenate itself.

In addition to acupuncture, herbal supplements provide another layer of support that can complement peptide therapy. Herbs like Ashwagandha and turmeric have been used for centuries to promote balance and vitality. When integrated with peptides, these natural supplements can enhance immune function, improve digestion, and support mental clarity. The combination of these therapies can create a comprehensive health regimen that addresses multiple aspects of wellness, from stress reduction to enhanced physical performance. For instance, Ashwagandha's adaptogenic properties help the body cope with stress, while turmeric's anti-inflammatory effects can enhance the body's healing processes. Together with peptides, these herbs can offer a multi-faceted approach to achieving optimal health.

Taking a multifaceted approach to health can yield benefits that surpass those of single therapies. By combining different modalities, you can address various facets of health, leading to enhanced recovery and improved mental well-being. Consider a scenario where peptides are used to accelerate muscle recovery post-exercise, while meditation is employed to reduce stress and promote relaxation. The peptides help repair tissues, while meditation calms the mind, reducing cortisol levels and fostering a state of balance. This integrated approach can lead to quicker recovery times and a more resilient body. Similarly, the use of herbal supplements alongside peptides can provide the necessary nutrients and support to sustain energy levels and enhance mental clarity throughout the day.

Let's explore a hypothetical example of a successful multi-therapy protocol. Imagine Jane, a professional dealing with high stress and chronic fatigue. She adopts a regimen that includes BPC-157 peptides for tissue repair, acupuncture sessions for stress relief, and a daily meditation practice. Over time, Jane notices a significant reduction in her fatigue levels and an improvement in her overall mood. The peptides help her body heal more efficiently, the acupuncture sessions release tension and improve energy flow, and meditation brings mental peace and clarity. This combination not only addresses her immediate concerns but also contributes to long-term health improvements, demonstrating the power of a comprehensive approach to wellness.

The potential of combining peptides with other therapies lies in the realm of exploration and experimentation. A spirit of curiosity is essential, as trying new wellness practices can lead to comprehensive and unexpected health improvements. Whether it's incorporating yoga for flexibility and relaxation or experimenting with dietary changes to support peptide efficacy, the possibilities are vast. Embrace the idea of trial and adaptation, knowing that everyone's path to wellness is unique. This willingness to explore different modalities can lead to discovering what works best for you, ultimately enhancing the benefits of peptide use. By remaining open to new ideas and approaches, you can craft a personalized health regimen that supports your goals and maximizes your potential for vitality and well-being.

The Ethical Considerations of Biohacking: Responsible Practices

As we venture into the domain of biohacking, particularly with the use of peptides, ethical considerations become paramount. Self-experimentation offers a pathway to individual health optimization, yet it raises profound moral questions. The autonomy to modify one's biology must be balanced with responsibility, ensuring that personal experimentation does not lead to harm. Consent in experimental contexts is crucial, especially when individuals share their experiences or involve others in their trials. Clear, informed consent respects autonomy and acknowledges the potential risks involved. It's not just about personal freedom; it's about making informed decisions that consider the broader impact on personal health and community standards.

Another layer of ethical consideration involves the sourcing and use of peptide materials. The demand for peptides has led to a burgeoning market, sometimes with murky sourcing practices. It's crucial to ensure that the peptides used are ethically sourced and adhere to standards that prioritize safety and efficacy. This requires diligence in choosing suppliers and a commitment to transparency about the origin and quality of the products. Ethical sourcing also involves considering the environmental impact of production processes, ensuring that the pursuit of personal health does not come at the expense of ecological well-being. It's about creating a balance where innovation thrives alongside ethical considerations.

Responsible biohacking hinges on informed decision-making and rigorous risk assessment. Understanding the potential risks versus the benefits of peptide use is crucial. While peptides can offer significant health benefits, they are not without risks, such as side effects or interactions with other medications. Consulting healthcare professionals before starting any peptide regimen is imperative.

These professionals provide valuable insights, ensuring that your approach to biohacking is both safe and effective. By making informed choices based on evidence and professional advice, you mitigate risks and enhance the likelihood of positive outcomes. This responsible approach underscores the importance of education and preparation in any biohacking endeavor.

The regulatory landscape surrounding peptide use adds another layer of complexity. Adhering to legal and ethical standards is not just a matter of compliance; it's a moral obligation. Navigating the regulatory requirements for peptide use involves understanding the laws governing their purchase and application. This includes ensuring that your use aligns with biohacking guidelines set by health authorities. Compliance ensures that you remain within legal boundaries, avoiding potential legal repercussions and contributing to a culture of accountability and integrity. It's about fostering an environment where innovation can flourish within ethical and legal frameworks.

Promoting a culture of safety and transparency is essential in the biohacking community. Open communication about results and experiences fosters a collaborative environment where knowledge is shared, and new insights are gained. Sharing your findings, whether successful or not, contributes to a collective understanding that benefits everyone. It encourages a community where ethical biohacking is the norm, and safety is prioritized. By fostering a transparent and supportive environment, we can collectively advance the field of biohacking, ensuring that it remains a force for good in the pursuit of health and wellness. This culture of openness and collaboration is key to navigating the complexities of biohacking responsibly.

In navigating these ethical considerations, we lay the groundwork for a responsible and sustainable approach to biohacking. The choices we make today set the stage for future developments, ensuring that the pursuit of health optimization remains aligned with the values of safety, integrity, and respect for all.

Conclusion

As we come to the end of our journey through the fascinating world of peptides, I want to take a moment to reflect on the path we've traveled together. From the very beginning, my goal has been to empower you with the knowledge and tools necessary to harness the incredible potential of these tiny molecules. We started by laying a solid foundation, exploring the basics of peptides and their role in the intricate dance of life within our bodies. Through vivid analogies and relatable examples, I aimed to demystify the science behind peptides, making it accessible to anyone with a passion for health optimization.

As we ventured deeper, we unraveled the mechanisms of action that make peptides such powerful agents of change. We discovered how they influence cellular communication, regulate biological processes, and offer targeted solutions for a wide range of health concerns. From enhancing muscle growth and repair to supporting cognitive function and longevity, the versatility of peptides became increasingly apparent with each chapter.

But this book is more than just a scientific exploration; it's a practical guide designed to help you integrate peptides into your own health journey. I've shared my expertise in crafting personalized peptide plans, emphasizing the importance of setting clear goals, understanding dosages and cycling, and monitoring progress. The real-world success stories peppered throughout the book serve as a testament to the transformative power of peptides when applied with knowledge and precision.

Conclusion

What sets this book apart is its commitment to providing a comprehensive resource that balances scientific depth with practical application. I've collaborated with leading experts in the field to bring you the latest insights and innovations, ensuring that you have access to the most up-to-date information available. From navigating the peptide marketplace to exploring advanced biohacking techniques, I've left no stone unturned in my quest to equip you with the tools you need to optimize your health.

But the journey doesn't end here. The world of peptides is constantly evolving, with discoveries and breakthroughs on the horizon. I encourage you to continue your exploration, armed with the knowledge and confidence you've gained from this book. Engage with the vibrant community of peptide enthusiasts, share your experiences, and learn from others who are passionate about biohacking. The connections you forge and the insights you gain will be invaluable as you refine your personalized approach to health optimization.

As you embark on this next phase of your journey, remember that the power to transform your health lies within you. The information and strategies outlined in this book are merely tools; it's up to you to wield them with wisdom and determination. Embrace the potential of peptides, but do so responsibly, always prioritizing safety and ethical considerations. The path to optimal health is not always easy, but with the right knowledge and mindset, it is undoubtedly achievable.

Conclusion

I want to express my heartfelt gratitude for joining me on this journey of discovery. Your commitment to learning and personal growth is truly inspiring. As someone who has witnessed firsthand the life-changing effects of peptides, I am thrilled to have had the opportunity to share my knowledge with you. Your success stories and transformations fuel my passion for this field and remind me of the incredible potential we all hold within us.

So, as you close this book and step forward into a world of endless possibilities, remember that you are now part of a community united by a shared vision of health and vitality. Continue to learn, grow, and inspire others with your own successes. Together, we can push the boundaries of what is possible and create a future where optimal health is within reach for all.

Thank you for embarking on this transformative journey with me. I can't wait to hear about your own peptide adventures and the incredible heights you'll reach. Here's to your health, your vitality, and the extraordinary potential that lies ahead!
With gratitude,
Asher Vale

HEALING WITH PEPTIDES:
THE ULTIMATE GUIDE TO BIOHACKING
YOUR BODY

HELP US GROW WITH YOUR REVIEW!

WE'D LOVE YOUR FEEDBACK!

THANK YOU FOR CHOOSING HEALING WITH PEPTIDES: THE ULTIMATE GUIDE TO BIOHACKING YOUR BODY AS PART OF YOUR HEALTH AND WELLNESS JOURNEY. YOUR FEEDBACK IS INCREDIBLY VALUABLE TO US! IF YOU FOUND THE INSIGHTS AND INFORMATION IN THIS BOOK HELPFUL, WE WOULD GREATLY APPRECIATE IT IF YOU COULD LEAVE A POSITIVE REVIEW. SIMPLY SCAN THE QR CODE BELOW TO SHARE YOUR THOUGHTS. YOUR REVIEW NOT ONLY SUPPORTS US IN REACHING MORE PEOPLE BUT ALSO HELPS TO SPREAD THE MESSAGE OF CUTTING-EDGE WELLNESS AND PEPTIDE-BASED HEALING.

THANK YOU FOR YOUR SUPPORT!

References

·What Is the Difference Between a Peptide and a Protein?
https://www.britannica.com/story/what-is-the-difference-between-a-peptide-and-a-protein#:~:text=The%20basic%20distinguishing%20factors%20are,50%20or%20more%20amino%20acids.

·Peptide Hormone - an overview
https://www.sciencedirect.com/topics/neuroscience/peptide-hormone

·Targeting peptide-mediated interactions in omics - PubMed
https://pubmed.ncbi.nlm.nih.gov/36461811/#:~:text=Peptide%2Dmediated%20interactions%20(PMIs),drug%20development%20and%20disease%20therapy.

·The Truth About Peptide Therapy: Debunking Common ...
https://klinic.com/blog/the-truth-about-peptide-therapy-debunking-common-myths-and-highlighting-key-facts-ltg7az1a

-Signaling Peptide - an overview | ScienceDirect Topics
https://www.sciencedirect.com/topics/biochemistry-genetics-and-molecular-biology/signaling-peptide#:~:text=The%20regulation%20of%20signaling%20pathways,or%20paracrine%20manner%20%5B1%5D.

·Capturing Peptide–GPCR Interactions and Their Dynamics
https://pmc.ncbi.nlm.nih.gov/articles/PMC7587574/#:~:text=Many%20biological%20functions%20of%20peptides,are%20a%20favorite%20pharmacological%20target.

·Dysregulation of Metabolic Peptides in the Gut–Brain Axis ...
https://www.mdpi.com/2227-9059/13/1/132#:~:text=Metabolic%20peptides%20such%20as%20GLP,expectancy%20by%205%E2%80%9310%20years.

·Effects of food-derived bioactive peptides on cognitive ...
https://www.sciencedirect.com/science/article/abs/pii/S0924224421004891
·Thymosin alpha 1: A comprehensive review of the literature
https://pmc.ncbi.nlm.nih.gov/articles/PMC7747025/
·The effects of human GH and its lipolytic fragment ...
https://pubmed.ncbi.nlm.nih.gov/11713213/
·Tesamorelin for GH Modulation and Fat Reduction
https://trtmd.com/tesamorelin-gh-modulation-fat-reduction/
·Treatment with the oral growth hormone secretagogue MK ...
https://pubmed.ncbi.nlm.nih.gov/9661080/
·Peptides for Muscle Growth https://marinregenhealth.com/peptide-therapy/peptides-for-muscle-growth/
·Essential Guide to Peptide Dosages: How to Safely ...
https://www.poseidonperformance.com/blog/essential-guide-to-peptide-dosages-how-to-safely-optimize-your-results
·Benefits & Risks of Peptide Therapeutics for Physical & ...
https://www.hubermanlab.com/episode/benefits-risks-of-peptide-therapeutics-for-physical-mental-health a comprehensive database of anti-aging peptides
https://pmc.ncbi.nlm.nih.gov/articles/PMC10930205/
-Regenerative and Protective Actions of the GHK-Cu ...
https://pmc.ncbi.nlm.nih.gov/articles/PMC6073405/
·6 Things to Know About Peptide Hormones and Releasing ...
https://www.usada.org/spirit-of-sport/6-things-know-peptide-hornes/
·Semax vs Noopept | What to Know in 2024
https://www.peptidesciences.com/peptide-research/semax-vs-noopept
· DSIP Peptide for Sleep https://www.transformyou.com/dsip
·Smart Sourcing for Peptides - by Katie Johnson
https://medium.com/@katiewritesfitness/smart-sourcing-for-peptides-5f28d3b7eafc
·Analysis of illegal peptide biopharmaceuticals frequently ...
https://pubmed.ncbi.nlm.nih.gov/26003685/
·Regulatory requirements of bioactive peptides (protein ...
https://www.sciencedirect.com/science/article/abs/pii/S1756464619302233l

·Peptide Storage and Handling Guidelines
https://www.genscript.com/peptide_storage_and_handling.html
·Understanding the Many Benefits of Peptide Therapy
https://modernaesthetica.com/biohacking-understanding-the-many-benefits-of-peptide-therapy/
·Editorial: Nutrigenomics and personalized nutrition
https://www.frontiersin.org/journals/nutrition/articles/10.3389/fnut.2024.1435475/full
·Therapeutic peptides: current applications and future ...
https://www.nature.com/articles/s41392-022-00904-4
·-Peptides for Athletes: A Comprehensive Guide
https://www.getphysical.com/blog/peptides-for-athletes-guide
·Therapeutic peptides: current applications and future ...
https://www.nature.com/articles/s41392-022-00904-4
· 101 – A New Deep Dive on Peptides with Expert, Ryan Smith
https://www.muscleintelligence.com/episode101/
·Peptides and Promises of Easy Recovery and Gains
https://www.quickanddirtytips.com/articles/peptides-and-promises-of-easy-recovery-and-gains/
·Journal of Peptide Science
https://onlinelibrary.wiley.com/journal/10991387